Religion
A Clinical Guide for Nurses

Elizabeth Johnston Taylor, PhD, RN, is an Associate Professor at the Loma Linda University School of Nursing, Loma Linda, CA. Dr. Taylor earned her MSN and PhD from the University of Pennsylvania and completed a postdoctoral fellowship at UCLA. She has received training in clinical pastoral education and spiritual direction. Dr. Taylor's program of research explores spiritual responses to illness and nurse-provided spiritual care. She has written over 70 publications, including 2 books on spiritual care. Currently, she serves on the editorial boards of the *Journal of Christian Nursing*, *Holistic Nursing Practice*, and *Home Healthcare Nurse*.

Religion

A Clinical Guide for Nurses

Elizabeth Johnston Taylor, PhD, RN
Editor

SPRINGER PUBLISHING COMPANY
NEW YORK

Springer Publishing Company, LLC
11 West 42nd Street
New York, NY 10036
www.springerpub.com
Acquisitions Editor: Margaret Zuccarini
Composition: The Manila Typesetting Company

ISBN: 978-0-8261-0860-9
E-book ISBN: 978-0-8261-0861-6

12 13 14/5 4 3 2 1

The author and the publisher of this work have made every effort to use sources believed to be reliable to provide information that is accurate and compatible with the standards generally accepted at the time of publication. The author and publisher shall not be liable for any special, consequential, or exemplary damages resulting, in whole or in part, from the readers' use of, or reliance on, the information contained in this book. The publisher has no responsibility for the persistence or accuracy of URLs for external or third-party Internet Web sites referred to in this publication and does not guarantee that any content on such Web sites is, or will remain, accurate or appropriate.

Library of Congress Cataloging-in-Publication Data
Religion : a clinical guide for nurses / [edited by] Elizabeth Johnston Taylor.
   p. ; cm.
Includes bibliographical references and index.
ISBN 978-0-8261-0860-9 — ISBN 978-0-8261-0861-6 (e-book)
I. Taylor, Elizabeth Johnston.
[DNLM: 1. Nurse's Role. 2. Religion and Medicine. 3. Spirituality. WY 87]

200.24'61073—dc23
                                                   2011051526

Special discounts on bulk quantities of our books are available to corporations, professional associations, pharmaceutical companies, health care organizations, and other qualifying groups. If you are interested in a custom book, including chapters from more than one of our titles, we can provide that service as well.

For details, please contact:
Special Sales Department, Springer Publishing Company, LLC
11 West 42nd Street, 15th Floor, New York, NY 10036-8002
Phone: 877-687-7476 or 212-431-4370; Fax: 212-941-7842
Email: sales@springerpub.com

Printed in the United States of America by Hamilton Printing

To my parents

Madeline S. and Robert M. Johnston

Who taught me health-promoting religion by modeling for me
how to dig roots deeply within a faith tradition
while maintaining a broader perspective, and
how to strive for a life where beliefs and practices are integrated and congruent.

Contents

Contributors

Muhamad Ali, PhD Assistant Professor in Islamic Studies, Religious Studies Department, University of California, Riverside, CA

Mark Carr, PhD Professor, School of Religion, Loma Linda University, Loma Linda, CA

The Reverend Peter Yuichi Clark, PhD Manager of Spiritual Care Services at UCSF Medical Center and UCSF Benioff Children's Hospital, San Francisco, and Associate Professor of Pastoral Care at the American Baptist Seminary of the West, Berkeley, CA

Shukavak Dasa, PhD Priest, Shri Lakshmi Narayan Mandir, Riverside, CA

Rabbi Elliot N. Dorff, PhD Distinguished Professor of Philosophy, American Jewish University, Los Angeles; Past President, Jewish Family Service of Los Angeles, Los Angeles, CA

Father Luke Dysinger, OSB, MD, DPhil Assistant Professor of Moral Theology and Church History, St. John's Seminary, Camarillo, CA

The Reverend Marsha D. M. Fowler, PhD, MDiv, MS, FAAN Professor, Azusa Pacific University, Azusa, CA

The Reverend David T. Gortner, MA, MDiv, PhD Professor of Evangelism and Congregational Leadership, and Director of Doctor of Ministry Programs, Virginia Theological Seminary, Alexandria, VA

Carol T. Kirk, RN, BSN, MS, CLNC Lark, High Priestess of the Oak, Ash, and Thorn Tradition of American Wicca; and Gardnerian Priestess, Ravenhurst Coven

Linda Kohler Christian Science nurse, and Manager, Christian Science Nursing Activities, The First Church of Christ, Scientist, Boston, MA

Joseph J. Kotva, Jr., PhD Executive Director, Anabaptist Center for Health Care Ethics, Associated Mennonite Biblical Seminary, Elkhart, IN

The Reverend John Luoma, PhD Visitation Pastor, Hope Lutheran Church, The Villages, FL, and formerly Professor of Historical Theology, Hamma School of Theology, Springfield, OH

Thomson K. Mathew, DMin, EdD Professor of Pastoral Care and Dean, College of Theology and Ministry, Oral Roberts University, Tulsa, OK

The Reverend John Matusiak, MDiv Media Coordinator, Orthodox Church in America, and Rector, St. Joseph Orthodox Christian Church, Wheaton, IL

Miguel Murillo Hospital Liaison Committee, Riverside, CA

The Reverend Susan Ritchie, PhD Professor of Unitarian Universalist History and Ministry, Starr King School for the Ministry, Graduate Theological Union, Berkeley, CA

Dennis Romain Chairman, Hospital Liaison Committee of Lower North Island, New Zealand

David Silverman President, American Atheists, Inc., Cranford, NJ

The Reverend Brenda Simonds, MDiv, BCC Director of Spiritual Care, Methodist Hospital of Southern California, Arcadia, CA

Pashaura Singh, PhD Professor and Dr. Jasbir Singh Saini Endowed Chair in Sikh and Punjabi Studies, Department of Religious Studies, University of California, Riverside, CA

The Reverend Joseph Smith Hospital Chaplain Endorser, Chaplain's Commission of IFCA International

Elizabeth Johnston Taylor, PhD, RN Associate Professor, School of Nursing, Loma Linda University, Loma Linda, CA

Tony Toneatto, PhD, CPsych Associate Professor, Department of Psychiatry, and Director, Buddhism, Psychology and Mental Health Minor Program, New College, University of Toronto, Toronto, Ontario, Canada

Brent L. Top, PhD Department Chair and Professor, Church History & Doctrine, Brigham Young University, Provo, UT

Lieutenant Justin B. Top Chaplain, U.S. Navy Naval Hospital, Jacksonville, FL

Reviewers

Lynn Callister, PhD, RN, FAAN   Professor Emerita, Brigham Young University, Provo, UT

Carl Christensen, PhD, RN   Dean, Buntain School of Nursing, Northwest University, Kirkland, WA

The Reverend Faye Davenport, RN, BA, BTh, MN, MEd   Senior Nursing Lecturer, Universal College of Learning; and Deacon, St. Peters Anglican Parish, Palmerston North, New Zealand

Anna Garton, RN   Mary Potter Hospice, Wellington, New Zealand

Russ Gerber   Christian Science Practitioner and Teacher, and Manager, Committees on Publication, Boston, MA

Patricia Gregory, RN   Staff Nurse, Northern California Eye Surgery Center, Citrus Heights, CA

Caz Haies, BNurs (Hons), PG Dip, RN   Lecturer in Clinical Nursing, Victoria University of Wellington, New Zealand

Marilyn Halstead, PhD, RN   Associate Professor Emeritus, Towson University, Towson, MD; Parish Nurse (Volunteer), First Presbyterian Church of Westminster, MD

Michael Hensley, RN   Kaiser Permanente, Calimesa, CA

Sharon T. Hinton, RN, MSN   Health Consultant, United Methodist Church General Board of Global Ministries, Floydada, TX

Harjit Kaur, MSocSc   Registered Clinical Counselor, Vancouver, British Columbia, Canada

Kathe Kelly, BSN, RN, OCN   City of Hope National Medical Center, Duarte, CA

Jacqueline Mickley, PhD, RN   Retired

Christina Miller, MS, MDiv, MA, RN   Nurse Coordinator for Palliative Care and Staff Chaplain, Sequoia Hospital, Redwood City, CA

Denise Miner-Williams, PhD, RN, CHPN   Research Assistant Professor, University of Texas Health Science Center, San Antonio School of Nursing, San Antonio, TX

Jessica Ongley, RN   Capital Coast District Health Board, Wellington, New Zealand

Eileen Schonfeld, BS ED, RN   Associate Chaplain, Akron General Medical Center; Volunteer Chaplain, Haslinger Pediatric Palliative Care Center, Akron Children's Hospital; and, Co-Director, Caring Community/Bikkur Cholim of Temple Israel, Akron, OH

Savitri W. Singh-Carlson, PhD, RN   Assistant Professor and Graduate Program Director, School of Nursing, California State University, Long Beach, CA

Rani Srivastava, PhD, RN   Chief of Nursing and Professional Practice, Centre for Addiction and Mental Health and Assistant Professor, Bloomberg Faculty of Nursing, University of Toronto, Toronto, Ontario, Canada

Rilla Taylor, EdD, RN   Adjunct Professor, Florida College of Health Sciences, Orlando, FL

Anna Frances Z. Wenger, PhD, RN, FAAN   Professor Emeritus, Goshen College, Goshen, IN

Preface

Whenever looking at nursing texts describing the health-related beliefs and practices of various religions, I naturally always have a look at how my own religion of Seventh-Day Adventism is portrayed. I can remember learning from these sources that I should give more credence to the Old Testament of the Christian Bible, rather than the New Testament. (Wrong.) I also read that my religion prohibited smoking, alcohol, and the eating of pork and that a vegetarian diet was prescribed. I never read about the diversity of diets members actually eat and how this often varies with the cultural background of the adherent. I read about the facts that make my religion stand out as different from others, but I never read about why that was. I never read about how people within my religious tradition think about suffering and cope with illness—cognitively or socially.

Because I found erroneous and essentialized information that was incomplete and misleading about my religion, I figured that that must be true for the other religions described in the nursing literature. This book offers an attempt to correct for this dearth of nursing-relevant information about religions. The information in this book can help nurses to avoid being negligent to patients whose religiosity overtly and covertly influences their responses to health-related challenges and transitions. Furthermore, this book—alongside its conceptually oriented companion by Marsha Fowler and colleagues, *Religion, Religious Ethics, and Nursing*—works to redress the damage done by the prevailing discourse in the nursing literature that disparages religion in favor of a generic spirituality. Yet this book does try to not blindly promote religiosity. It recognizes its potential for harm as well as for good in the health care arena.

The focal point of this book is the splendid collection of 22 contributions from religionists who are not only experts about a faith tradition but also adherents of it (Section II). These contributions were generated by a list of around 20 questions that were posed to each contributor. After compiling these responses, I identified what I thought might be the nursing implications unique for each tradition. To increase the validity of these pieces, nurses who likewise were adherents of these respective religions reviewed them to ensure accuracy and appropriateness of the contents for nursing.

Section I chapters that precede the contributions describing various religions offer context and guidance for clinical practice. An explanation on why patient religiosity is important for nurses to support is found in Chapter 1, as well as some brief contextual background about what religion is. Chapter 2 provides information about how to talk with patients about religion, a fundamental skill for respecting the religiosity of patients and their loved ones. Following on these communication skills is Chapter 3, which offers information about how to assess religiosity. Because religion at the bedside often manifests in overt rituals, Chapter 4 addresses how nurses can support such rituals. To ethically and legally integrate this information in clinical care, Chapters 5 and 6 offer legal and ethical perspectives, respectively. Because ethical nursing care in this regard requires an awareness of self and how personal religiosity (or lack thereof) influences caring, Chapter 7 provides discussion and opportunity for reflection about how a nurse's religiosity inevitably has an impact on nursing practice.

Acknowledgments

Supporting me through this endeavor were family, friends, and even acquaintances I have never met in person. It warms the "cockles of my heart" to thank these gracious persons. This book is a product of collegial work with my friends and mentors who provided wonderful insights as this book began: Marsha Fowler, Barb Pesut, Sheryl Reimer-Kirkham, and Rick Sawatzky. I am also grateful to lawyers Roger Lang and Laura Fry, who helped me when I ventured into what for me was previously uncharted waters: legal perspectives about religion in nursing care. The feat of finding religionist contributors and nurse reviewers to represent 22 traditions took some effort. I am most grateful to numerous individuals who made this possible, including but not limited to Jackie Mickley, Kathy Schoonover-Shoffner, Kathy McMillan, and Larry Swinford. My "bosses" Marilyn Herrmann (Loma Linda University, Loma Linda, CA) and Brian Ensor (Mary Potter Hospice, Wellington, Aotearoa New Zealand) have supported this effort by kindly granting me flexibility with time. I am also deeply appreciative to Springer's nursing publisher, Margaret Zuccarini, who warmly welcomed me to the Springer fold and has always given me good counsel. Finally, I want to thank my husband, Lyndon, and daughters, Elissa Lynn and Rilla Kathryn, for their sacrifices that have allowed me to complete this personally satisfying project.

Religion
A Clinical Guide for Nurses

Religion and Nursing Care

INTRODUCTION

A New York City-based clinical nurse specialist was having serious complications from major abdominal surgery. She was physically and emotionally exhausted and anxious about not healing. Being Jewish, she thought having her nurse pray for her would be comforting. She was, however, very nervous about asking for prayer. She pondered for some time whether she should ask the nurse. Then, she pondered how she should ask the nurse. When her nurse next came to her bedside (to change an intravenous fluid), my acquaintance asked: "Um, if—if—it is okay with you, would you mind saying a prayer for me?" Her longing for spiritual sustenance and hopeful expectations for finding such with the aid of the nurse were dashed when the nurse appeared to look uncomfortable and stated, "I don't do that." The nurse quickly finished her task and left this bedside opportunity.

Contrasting true stories exist (Taylor, 2011). An English nurse was suspended from her duties because she asked a patient if she would appreciate a prayer at the end of a short home care visit to provide wound care. This recipient of care told the nursing agency that although she did not mind being asked, she thought this nurse's religious offer could be upsetting to others. A Massachusetts nurse was similarly relieved of duties when she engaged a dying patient with AIDS in a discussion about repentance. This patient's family reported that he had been distraught by this conversation.

These stories raise many questions. Should nurses ever offer religious "interventions" at the bedside? Is it right—or possible, or even helpful—for a nurse to respond to any patient's religious queries or needs? If so, under what circumstances? Why, when, and how should a nurse address or support patient religiosity in a therapeutic and ethical manner?

These three stories also raise questions about the role of a nurse's personal spiritual or religious beliefs in providing patient care. Can a nurse's religiosity (or nonreligiosity) be surgically removed while on duty? If not, how ought a nurse's personal spiritual or religious beliefs influence his or her nursing care? In addition to questions of ethics about introducing religion into the nurse–patient encounter, what are the legal boundaries for doing so?

These stories also illustrate the clinical reality of how religious practices and talk are sometimes comforting and appreciated by patients and sometimes discomforting and disconcerting to patients. Why might religious beliefs or practices be sometimes helpful and sometimes harmful? What mechanisms explain health-promoting or health-demoting religious beliefs and practices?

These questions are necessary to answer if a nurse is to give spiritually and culturally sensitive holistic care. The next seven chapters offer answers to these questions. The contextual information and clinical guidance these chapters provide will allow you to provide nursing care in this regard that is ethical, legal, and therapeutic.

REFERENCE

Taylor, E. J. (2011). Spiritual care: Evangelism at the bedside? *Journal of Christian Nursing, 28*(4), 194–202.

Religion at the Bedside: Why?

Elizabeth Johnston Taylor, PhD, RN

Religion typically is a taboo topic. Why should nurses risk embarrassment to broach the subject? For what reason should they bother to recognize religiosity in patients or in themselves?

Consider these scenarios: A Hindu wants her teeth brushed *before* breakfast. A Sikh preparing for surgery is distraught that his hair will be shaved. An atheist or neopagan patient may loathe having a chaplain visit. An Amish declines to make a treatment decision without consulting and praying with fellow believers. A bed-bound Muslim asks you for support to say daily prayers. A Buddhist is wishful about not being able to chant. A nurse colleague refuses to provide care for a patient because of a conscientious objection. Another coworker offers prayer to all her patients. Why? How do you respond ethically, legally, and therapeutically to such queries and circumstances?

Throughout this book, it is argued that when religion interacts with health and illness, it is requisite to effective and ethical nursing care to recognize this religion–health relationship. This chapter will review research and theory linking religion and health. This review provides a context and foundation for the ensuing chapters that propose how the nurse can provide religion-sensitive care.

REASONS FOR RECOGNIZING RELIGION IN PATIENT CARE

A number of reasons support why nurses should appreciate the role of religion as they provide health care.

Many Patients Are Religious

Whether caring for a patient from a first- or third-world country, it is more likely than not that they are religious. Furthermore, although this is a point that would be inappropriate to push, even nonreligious persons are often influenced by the religion of their parents or other sources of authority and society. Census data from English-speaking first-world countries indicate that the majority of people do identify themselves as religious. Conversely, self-reported nonreligiosity in the largest of these countries falls within a small and narrow range of 15%–18% (Department of Immigration and Citizenship, 2008; Kosmin & Keysar, 2008; National Statistics, 2010; Statistics Canada, 2001). Religiosity appears to be greater among older rather than young adults, greater among women than men, and greater among African Americans and Latinos than Asians and those of European descent (Pew Forum, 2010a). Although a large majority of citizens report a religious affiliation, this does not mean they deem religion as important. In a Gallup (2010) survey of Americans, 56% believed religion was very important in their own life, whereas 25% believed it was fairly important, and 19% thought it was not very important. Likewise, 65% said religion was an important "part of daily life."

Several recent trends have been observed in these countries. One is a trend in the movement from religious affiliation to none. While some "nones" are atheist or agnostic, many are simply "nothing in particular." Indeed, an American survey found that of the 5% who do not believe in a God or universal spirit, only 24% called themselves atheist (Pew Forum, 2010b). Another trend is the increase in non-Christian adherents, which reflects immigration patterns. While Christianity remains the dominant world faith in these countries, there have been steady increases in the numbers of non-Christians, particularly among Muslims and Hindus (e.g., Statistics Canada, 2001). Although only 4% of the American population affiliates with a non-Christian religion, this group grew 50% between 1990 and 2008 (Kosmin & Keysar, 2008). Even within Christianity, there has been a shifting away from the historic mainline churches to evangelical and nondenominational churches (Kosmin & Keysar). Among religious Americans, there is also an increase in the mixing of multiple faiths (e.g., "hyphenated Christians"). For example, 35% of Americans occasionally or regularly attend services of a different tradition from their own. This mixing and matching of beliefs often involves mixing Christian beliefs with Eastern or New Age beliefs (Pew Forum, 2009).

Religiosity Is Associated With Health Outcomes

Research examining the relationships between aspects of religiosity and health generally (but not always) show positive linkages. Whether it is frequency of attendance at religious services, use of meditational prayer, high intrinsic religiosity, or some other indicator of religiosity, findings suggest that these indicators of religiosity associate with or predict health outcomes such as mortality, morbidity, adjustment to illness, and quality of life (e.g., Koenig, McCullough, & Larson, 2001; Levin, 2001).

Levin (2001) asserts six mechanisms for explaining how religiosity can contribute to good health. These include:

- *Religious proscriptions that support healthful lifestyles and behaviors.* For example, most religious traditions advocate that sexual intercourse be confined to a committed, covenanted, and monogamous relationship; this behavior, if adhered to, eliminates the possibility of sexually transmitted disease. Most religions also denigrate the abuse of alcohol or nontherapeutic substances. Observant and conservative members of several religious traditions will respect proscriptions about food (e.g., Jews, Buddhists, Hindus, Muslims). These proscriptions, although varied, generally endorse ways of eating that are now understood to be healthful (e.g., vegetarian, not overindulging, avoiding meat with higher potential for disease). Epidemiological research has demonstrated Latter-Day Saints and Seventh-Day Adventists, who characteristically observe many of these health proscriptions, do live longer (Koenig et al., 2001).

- *Regular religious fellowship that benefits health by offering support that buffers the effects of stress and isolation.* For many who remain in a religious organization, it is the sense of belonging that may keep them affiliated. A faith community is like an extended family for many. Furthermore, within a society, a faith community often affords persons from different social strata an opportunity to equalize with those from higher and lower strata. This mechanism for obtaining social support allows isolated and marginalized—and healthy—individuals a structure for social safety, a place to weep and laugh with others, to give and take comfort, to belong. Although any family may have its "warts," such a community typically offers social support. Krause and Ellison's (2009) findings extend this assertion further. They observed that congregants who had negative encounters in their parish were more likely to have religious doubt and that suppressing doubts about religion was associated with poorer health. In contrast, congregants who attended a Bible study group (i.e., obtained better social support) were more apt to look for spiritual growth in response to a situation that raised religious doubt.

- *Participation in worship and prayer that benefits health through the physiological effects of positive emotions.* There has been considerable empirical effort during the past decade to explore the mechanisms that could explain the linkage between neurobiology and religiosity (Griffith, 2010). While much mystery exists about the biology of belief, it is known that worshipful experiences often create some degree of ecstasy, which in turn creates a physical state of well-being. Similarly, prayer can (but not always) contribute to an inner state of peace or joy. Such positive feelings of deep contentment or understanding affect body chemistry, stimulating health-promoting molecules of emotion and affecting physical well-being. Offering a glimpse into this process is a clever study done by Wiech et al. (2008) that allowed functional magnetic resonance imaging (fMRI) to compare the perceived intensity of induced pain on Roman Catholics looking at a picture of the Virgin Mary with that of nonreligious subjects looking at a da Vinci picture of the "Woman with Ermine." The Catholic subjects perceived significantly less pain and were observed to have increased activation of the right ventrolateral prefrontal cortex, known to be activated during times of cognitive control over pain.

- *Simple faith that benefits health by leading to thoughts of hope, optimism, and positive expectation.* For instance, most religions offer a way of making sense of why bad things happen to people, even good people (i.e., theodicies). Most religions also give believers hope in an afterlife. Many religions also provide a way of thinking about death that reframes the death in a positive light (e.g., death is sleep that ends at a second advent of Jesus, death allows the soul to go to heaven and be with God, death is a rebirth to a better existence).

- *Mystical experiences that benefit health by activating a healing bioenergy, or life force, or altered state of consciousness.* Whether it is a meditational state, a physically induced ecstasy (e.g., from religious dance or music or hallucinogenic substance), or a unitive moment (i.e., transient, random, experience of awareness of something greater or exceptional insight), esoteric religious experiences are accompanied by a sense of meaningfulness, happiness, and feeling of well-being.

- *Divine intervention that allows healing.* Although the divine is ultimately mysterious, and it is inappropriate and impossible to adequately test this assertion (Cohen, Wheeler, Scott, Edwards, Lusk, et al., 2000), many religious believers accept that the divine is omnipotent and involved with individuals in personal and intimate ways. Interpretations about how the divine intervenes in human life and earthly circumstances, of course, vary with religious tradition. Some believe that miracles continually occur as a natural result of divine laws of nature, while others accept that the divine can purposefully affect these laws to intervene and cause a magical miracle. This is illustrated in a case study of a woman with Huntington's disease who visited Lourdes and perceived that the Virgin Mary spoke to her, telling her that she was cured (Moreno & de Yebenes, 2009). Although she continued to take her medicine, this woman was ecstatic about her "miraculous cure." In subsequent examinations by two experts, a nearly complete elimination of dystonia and chorea were observed along with a 40% improvement (using a standardized score), but no cure genetically. These neurologists conjectured a placebo effect accounted for the "cure," perhaps related to the known direct relationship between anxiety and chorea (Moreno & de Yebenes). Indeed, diverse views of divine intervention can produce varying perspectives such as "without medicine, God can cure me of my illness," to "using natural pathways yet unknown, God can cure me," or "using the miracle of human knowing about medicine, God can cure me of my illness." Others may simply accept that "whether I survive cancer or not, the miracle is that I have been given breath today."

These conjectures about how religion affects health suggest that religiosity is an important topic for nurses interested in health promotion and illness management.

Religious Beliefs Influence Health Decision Making

One's religious beliefs can guide decision making by providing "an interpretive framework that helps to move forward in the face of overwhelming and intelligible circumstances" (White, 2009, p. 75). The growing body of evidence linking religious belief with health care decision making describes the influence of beliefs on varied decisions, from those related to pregnancy and genetic testing to cancer and HIV treatment (Taylor, 2011). Most of the research, however, illuminates how beliefs impact end-of-life-related decisions, such as those around resuscitation and prolongation of life and advanced directives and elder care planning.

Religions Offer Coping Strategies

Until around the turn of the century, health-related research documenting religious coping often did so by framing it in behavioral terms. That is, this research described how patients used prayer, reading holy writings, devotional and other religious practices to cope with illness (Taylor, 2002). (While many religious persons would argue that their practices are not used magically to gain outcomes, this may be true for some.) These religious coping strategies often buffer stress and provide much emotional comfort for believers.

More recently, however, this area of study is influenced by Pargament's conceptualization of religious coping as comprising positive and/or negative beliefs (Pargament, Koenig, & Perez, 2000). Ano and Vasconcelles' (2005) meta-analysis of 49 investigations exploring the relationship between religious coping and psychological adjustment to stress concluded that, in general, positive religious coping was associated with adjustment. Conversely, negative religious coping was associated with poor adjustment. This evidence calls nurses to support positive religious coping and consider how to address the deleterious effects of negative religious coping when it impacts health (Taylor, 2011).

Religious Beliefs and Practices May Have Health Implications

As this book will unpack, religious persons may practice rituals that have physical or mental health implications. These could include pilgrimages, ascetic practices, diets, "complementary" therapies, or other practices. Likewise, a religious patient will have religious beliefs about what causes illness, how to respond to suffering, what is life and death, and so forth. These beliefs will inevitably influence the way religious patients take care of their health. Furthermore, a health-related event may have religious

implications (e.g., a Hindu discharged from a hospitalization may participate in a ritual that symbolizes purification).

Some Patients Want Nurses to Support Their Religiosity

A few studies have surveyed patients about whether they would want
their nurse to inquire about and be respectful of their spirituality and religion. While most patients do want clinicians to know about their spirituality, they do not view them as primary spiritual caregivers. Religious
persons, as well as those who are experiencing life-threatening conditions,
are especially eager for a nurse to discuss with them how best to support
their religiosity (Taylor, 2007; Taylor & Mamier, 2005).

Professional Mandates

The Joint Commission (2008), the accrediting body from which most U.S.
health care organizations seek approval, mandates that all patients receive a
spiritual assessment. The Joint Commission recognizes religion as a salient
aspect of a patient spirituality and advises that religion is to be respected
and supported. Likewise, various nursing codes for ethical conduct specifically identify the religiosity of patients as a dimension of personhood the
nurse must respect (see Chapter 6, Nursing Codes of Ethics).

Further endorsement for recognizing the salience of religion in nursing
comes from NANDA International, which categorizes religious problems
and strengths with diagnostic labels (Gordon, 2007). Although these diagnostic labels exist, nurses must be cautious about pathologizing patient
religiosity. That is, although some religious problems may be unhealthful,
religious distress can also be indicative of healthful spiritual maturation—
spiritual growing pains perhaps. For example, a "dark night of the soul"
is not depression, rather a spiritual dryness the person knows to be a gift
that expands one's understanding of God.

THEORIES ABOUT RELIGION

During the last half of the 19th century, social scientists began formally
theorizing about how religions originate and function in society. Varied
theories arose (Pals, 2006). For example, Freud portrayed religion as wish
fulfillment resulting from neuroses. Marx viewed religion as a way of coping with class struggle. Others saw religion as a cultural system of symbols played out in beliefs and practices that create community or social
cohesion (e.g., Durkheim, Geertz). Another theory about religion posits
that it is economically driven; that is, religious beliefs that bring about
advantages are chosen (Stark & Finke). Others have proposed that religious beliefs about the divine are anthropomorphic; that is, in response
to ambiguity, humans project human attributes on nonhuman entities to
create a personal god (Guthrie, 2007).

Social scientists also describe facets of religion with typologies. For example, Glock and Stark (1965) propose that religions have five dimensions: doctrinal, intellectual, ethical, private devotional and public ritual, and experiential. Wallace (1966) describes the typical components of religion as prayer (addressing the supernatural); music and artistic expression; physical manipulation of one's psychological state; exhortation or addressing other humans (e.g., sermons); reciting the religion's code or aspects of belief or history; touching that transfers supernatural power through contact; taboo or not touching certain things; simulation or imitating things; feasts; sacrifice (e.g., offerings); congregation; and inspiration (i.e., recognizing the divine in human experience). Troeltsch (1991) describes the primary types of religions. He suggests three: religious organizations that are inclusive and accommodate societal institutions; sects that demand voluntary commitment of members, are perfectionistic, and critical of the social milieu; and mysticism (an individual, spiritual religiosity).

Several religionists also offer theories about how religions evolve. Older theories describe progressive stages of organized religiosity (e.g., from individualistic and shamanistic religion to communal and collective to monotheistic and ecclesiastical) (Wallace, 1966). The recent trend, however, is to explain sociobiologically how religion exists in humans. This theorizing is informed by neurobiological science and psychology. One theory that has failed to receive further support is that there is a "God gene" that biologically explains why some people are religious (Pals, 2006). Currently, there is debate about whether research using fMRI that shows brain activity during religious experiences to be like the activity found during other human experiences (e.g., intimate interpersonal relating, cognitive coping) actually proves that religiosity is a by-product of culture or manifestation of how the human species adapts (e.g., Fingelkurts & Fingelkurts, 2009; Thomson & Aukofer, 2011).

Although some would argue that religiosity is irrational—a hijacking of the human mind or result of evolutionary misfiring (Thomson & Aukofer, 2011), all would agree that humans are very vulnerable to religious belief. Those who believe their religious experience is a result of a supernatural creative Entity, of course, can still accept that no matter how their religious experience manifests biologically in association with other cognitive processes, this vulnerability to belief is nevertheless valid and a gift allowing relationship with the divine.

Regardless, the sociobiological systems innate in humans do play an important role in religious behavior (Griffith, 2010), whether they explain religion as a by-product of adaptation or not. These systems for which humans are wired include:

- Attachment or the need to feel safe and close to a secure attachment figure (e.g., manifested in religious statements such as "God is my loving Father")

- Peer affiliation or the need for feeling safe and part of a cohesive group, such as a faith community

- Kin recognition or having tradition-specific attributes and rituals that separate and unify adherents (e.g., dress, holy days, labels for religious kin like "brother," "sister," "elder")

- Social hierarchy (e.g., for theists, the ultimate "alpha male" is God; local congregations have some stratification of members)

- Social exchange and reciprocal altruism that assures the believer that ultimately life will be good and fair (e.g., righteousness will be rewarded with a blissful afterlife, evil will be condemned at a final judgment).

These systems indeed allow humans to adapt to life's challenges and protect our species.

Social scientists have theorized that religion will die due to modernization and secularization. This prediction, however, continues to be disproved (Hefner, 2009). While in some areas of the world ecclesiastical religion may be declining, overall, there has been an increase in religiosity globally. Religion, regardless of its causal factors, appears here to stay.

RELIGION DEFINED

Although over a century of scientific study of religion from the perspective of multiple disciplines has produced numerous theories, there is no one commonly used definition of religion. The definition accepted for this discussion about religion in patient care is that offered by Hill et al. (2000):

> The feelings, thoughts, experiences, and behaviors that arise from a search for the sacred. The term "search" refers to attempts to identify, articulate, maintain, or transform. The term "sacred" refers to a divine being, divine object, Ultimate Reality, or Ultimate Truth as perceived by the individual. (p. 66)

This definition contains the criteria for spirituality. To define religion, Hill et al. suggest this definition of spirituality must be extended to also include or instead be "A search for non-sacred goals (such as identity, belongingness, meaning, health, or wellness) in a context that has as its primary goal the facilitation of [the above criterion for spirituality]" and "the means and methods (e.g., rituals or prescribed behaviors) of the search that receive validation and support from within an identifiable group of people" (p. 66). Thus, religion involves individuals seeking that which is ultimately sacred using prescribed means endorsed by a group.

Whereas the concept now labeled "spirituality" was until relatively recently considered an aspect of religion, most academics now distinguish spirituality from religion. Indeed, this distinction between spirituality and religion is now common in the general public. Indeed, a few studies have documented that while the majority of Americans self-define as spiritual and religious, a substantial minority view themselves as spiritual but not religious (Grant, O'Neill, & Stephens, 2003; Zinnbauer et al., 1997). Although religion is typically thought of as institutional and objective while the very elastic and generic term spirituality is individual and subjective, these two concepts are deeply intertwined (Hill et al., 2000).

A CAVEAT: WHEN RELIGION HARMS

The evidence referenced above indicates that, overall, religion is good for one's health. This, however, is not always true. If the product of religiosity is confusion, despair, isolation, helplessness, meaninglessness, detachment, or resentment, then that religiosity is causing harm (Griffith, 2010).

Pargament and others differentiate between religious coping that is positive or is negative (Ano & Vasconcelles, 2005; Pargament, Koenig, & Perez, 2000). Negative religious coping is exemplified by Demonic reappraisals (e.g., "Decided the devil made this happen"), reappraisal of God's power (e.g., "Realized that God cannot answer all my prayers"), passive religious deferral (e.g., "Didn't do much, just expected God to solve my problems for me"), and pleading for direct intercession (e.g., "Prayed for a miracle"). Thus, when a religious person holds beliefs that are not assuring or comforting, create unhelpful guilt or shame, instill passivity, or create a sense of abandonment, this is not healthful. Numerous studies have documented that such negative religious coping is correlated with poor adjustment during health challenges (Ano & Vasconcelles).

Griffith (2010), a Christian psychiatrist, offers an in-depth explanation about how religion can become harmful or healing. Griffith asserts that religion becomes harmful when one of three core roles of religion is prioritized over the others, diminishing personal spirituality (or "whole person relatedness"). That is, if any one of the roles of religion to ensure group security, strengthen the adherent's sense of worth, or ease personal suffering becomes significantly more important to the believer than are the other two roles, then religion becomes harmful. Such imbalance is manifested then in religiosity that contributes to suffering, such as when one experiences the divine as an insecure attachment figure, when one searches for security primarily within a religious group, when one accepts religious beliefs to the exclusion of any alternative beliefs, or when a religious group protects only their own. Mental illness can also undermine religious experience. Griffith identifies how religious beliefs can be the vehicle expressing mental illness. Mood disorders, anxiety, and psychoses can distort religious experience as well.

Ultimately, religion becomes harmful when personal spirituality becomes diminished or dies (Griffith, 2010). Healthy personal spirituality involves: a whole person relatedness or "I/thou" relationship with the divine; personal encounters with the sacred that stimulate creativity, reflection, and moral thinking; a dedication to being compassionate toward others and oneself; resilience; and an ability to prioritize the well-being of self and others over those of the religious group. Griffith's observations confirm what some research indicates as well: It is a combination of positive religiosity and intrinsic personal spirituality that may be most adaptive and healthful (Taylor, 2011).

PRIMARY PRACTICE POINTS

- Research evidence indicates direct associations between religion and health.

- Nurses have many reasons for recognizing patient religiosity. These include the fact that religion is prevalent, that some religious practices have health-related implications, and that some health-related events have religious implications for adherents of some religions, and professional mandates.

- Religion serves many functions, from social cohesion to intrapsychic comfort.

- When religion lacks personal spirituality (whole person relatedness), it becomes harmful.

REFERENCES

Ano, G., & Vasconcelles, E. (2005). Religious coping and psychological adjustment to stress: A meta-analysis. *Journal of Clinical Psychology, 61*, 461–480.

Cohen, C. B., Wheeler, S. E., Scott, D. A., Edwards, B. S., Lusk, P., & the Anglican Working Group in Bioethics. (2000). Prayer as therapy: A challenge to both religious beliefs and professional ethics. *Hastings Center Report, 30*, 40–47.

Department of Immigration and Citizenship. (2008). *The people of Australia: Statistics from the 2006 census*. Retrieved February 28, 2010, from http://www.immi.gov.au/media/publications/research/_pdf/poa-2008.pdf

Fingelkurts, A. A., & Fingelkurts, A. A. (2009). Is our brain hardwired to produce God, or is our brain hardwired to perceive God? A systematic review on the role of the brain in mediating religious experience. *Cognitive Processing, 10*(4), 293–326.

Gallup. (2011). *Religion*. Retrieved March 2, 2011, from http://www.gallup.com/poll/1690/Religion.aspx

Glock, C. Y., & Stark, R. (1965). *Religion and society in tension*. Chicago, IL: Rand McNally.

Gorden, M. (2010). *Manual of nursing diagnosis* (12th ed.). Sudbury, MA: Jones & Bartlett.

Grant, D., O'Neil, K. M., & Stephens, L. S. (2003). Neosecularization and craft versus professional religious authority in a nonreligious organization. *Journal for the Scientific Study of Religion, 43*, 479–487.

Griffith, J. L. (2010). *Religion that heals, religion that harms*. New York, NY: Guilford.

Guthrie, S. E. (2007). Opportunity, challenges and a definition of religion. *Journal for the Scientific Study of Religion, Nature, & Culture, 1*, 58–67.

Hefner, R. W. (2009). Religion and modernity worldwide. In P. B. Clark (Ed.). *The Oxford handbook of the sociology of religion* (pp. 152–167). New York, NY: Oxford University Press.

Hill, P. C., Pargament, K. I., Hood, R. W., Jr., McCullough, M. E., Swyers, J. P., Larson, D. B., et al. (2000). Conceptualizing religion and spiritualty: Points of commonality, points of departure. *Journal for the Theory of Social Behavior, 30*(1), 51–77.

Joint Commission. (2008). *Comprehensive accreditation manual for hospitals: The official handbook*. Oakbrook Terrace, IL: Author.

Koenig, H. G., McCullough, M. E., & Larson, D. B. (2001). *Handbook of religion and health*. Oxford, UK: Oxford University Press.

Kosmin, B. A., & Keysar, A. (2009). *American Religious Identification Survey 2008*. Retrieved March 3, 2009, from http://wwwamericanreligioussurvey-aris.org/reports/ARIS_Report_2008.pdf

Krause, N. & Ellison, C. G. (2009). The doubting process: A longitudinal study of the precipitants and consequences of religious doubt. *Journal for the Scientific Study of Religion, 48*, 293–312.

Levin, J. S. (2001). *God, faith, and health: Exploring the spirituality–healing connection*. New York, NY: Wiley.

Moreno, J. L., & de Yebenes, J. G. (2009). The impact of an intense religious experience on motor symptoms in Huntington's Disease. *Movement Disorders, 24*, 473–474.

National Statistics. (2004). *Religion: Religious populations*. Retrieved February 28, 2010, from http://www.statistics.gov.uk/cci/nugget_print.asp?ID=954

Pals, D. L. (2006). *Eight theories of religion* (2nd ed.). New York, NY: Oxford University Press.

Pargament, K., Koenig, H., & Perez, L. (2000). The many methods of religious coping: Development and validation of the RCOPE. *Journal of Clinical Psychology, 56*, 519–543.

Pew Forum on Religion and Public Life. (2009). *Many Americans mix multiple faiths*. Retrieved May 8, 2011, from http://pewforum.org/docs/?DocID=490

Pew Forum on Religion and Public Life. (2010a). *Belief in God*. Retrieved May 8, 2011, from http://www.pewforum.org/Age/Religion-Among-the-Millenials.aspx

Pew Forum on Religion and Public Life. (2010b). *Not all nonbelievers call themselves atheists*. Retrieved May 9, 2011, from http://www.pewforum.org/Not-All-Nonbelievers-Call-Themselves-Atheists.aspx?print=true

Pew Forum on Religion and Public Life. (2011). *U.S. Religious landscape survey: Affiliations*. Retrieved May 8, 2011, from http://www.religions.pewforum.org/affiliations

Statistics Canada. (n. d.). *Selected religions, for Canada, provinces and territories—20 sample data*. Retrieved February 28, 2010, from http://www12.statcan.ca/english/census01/products/highlight/Religion/PrintFriendly.cfm

Taylor, E. J. (2007). *What do I say? Talking with patients about spirituality*. Philadelphia, PA: Templeton Press.

Taylor, E. J. (2011). Religion and patient care. In M. D. Fowler, S. Reimer-Kirkham, R. Sawatzky, & E. J. Taylor (Eds.), *Religion, religious ethics, and nursing* (pp. 313–338). New York, NY: Springer Publishing Company.

Taylor, E. J., & Mamier, I. (2005). Spiritual care nursing: What cancer patients and family caregivers want. *Journal of Advanced Nursing, 49*(3), 260–267.

Thomson, J. A., & Aukofer, C. (2011). *Why we believe in God(s)*. Charlottesville, VA: Pitchstone.

Troeltsch, E. (1991). *Religion in history*. Minneapolis, MN: Fortress Press.

Wallace, A. F. C. (1966). *Religion: An anthropological view*. New York, NY: Random House.

White, M. T. (2009). Making sense of genetic uncertainty: The role of religion and spirituality. *American Journal of Medical Genetics, Part C, Seminars in Medical Genetics, 151C*(1), 68–76.

Wiech, K., Farias, M., Kahane, G., Shackel, N., Tiede, W., Tracy, I., et al. (2008). An fMRI study measuring analgesia enhanced by religion as a belief system. *Pain, 139,* 467–476.

Zinnbauer, B. J., Pargament, K. I., Cole, B. C., Rye, M. S., Butter, E. M., Belavich, T. G., et al. (1997). Religion and spirituality: Unfuzzying the fuzzy. *Journal for the Scientific Study of Religion, 36,* 549–564.

2 Talking With Patients About Religion

Elizabeth Johnston Taylor, PhD, RN

What do I do when a religious patient is trying to convert me? Sometimes I feel like I am not very good at listening to a patient who uses a lot of religious language and ideas. How can I be a better listener for religious patients who push my buttons? Or perhaps, you are a religious nurse, and you are wondering how you can discreetly introduce your comforting beliefs to patients while you are conversing with them? Regardless of which question you may be asking, this chapter will present principles and practice suggestions that address these sticky questions.

PRINCIPLES

While it is advisable to consider whether discussing religion with a patient is legal under your circumstances, it is more important to ask if it is ethical. As Chapter 6 on Ethical Perspectives discusses, a nurse should only talk about religion if the patient introduces it or if it is necessary for reasons related to nursing and health care. Given both of these conditions often present, let us explore how to respectfully engage in nurse–patient discourse involving religion.

Goals for Conversation About Religiosity

This chapter's discussion about how to talk with patients about religiosity assumes the purpose of the talk is for therapeutic purposes other than assessment. It is often true, however, that during nurse–patient conversations, assessment data is also obtained (see Chapter 3). Whether a nurse assesses that talking about the patient's religiosity is necessary for quality health care or because a patient introduces the topic, the principles of empathic communication advanced by psychologists should shape the therapeutic discourse. Because most nurses have limited time and training to offer a patient counseling, an appropriate goal for nurse–patient discourse about spiritual or religious matters is to allow the patient to simply explore their concerns (Taylor, 2007a). This exploration can lead, even if incrementally, the patient to gain insight and problem solve. If the goal for the nurse–patient discourse about religion is not to assess, then it is to support the patient in exploring how their religiosity and well-being intersect. To adapt Taylor's goal for clinicians who talk with patients about spirituality, the goal here is to support the patient to become more aware

15

of their religious experience and how it impacts health so that they can experience life more fully.

Guidelines for Communication About Religiosity

The following guidelines (Burleson, 2003; Taylor, 2007a) are vital to observe when talking with a patient about religiosity:

- Be nondirective (versus authoritarian). This means not giving advice and interpretations, not controlling or dominating the conversation. (This is especially challenging when the patient's religiosity appears illogical, never mind harmful.) For example, if a distraught patient says she questions "if there is a God out there for me," an appropriate answer might be, "Tell me more about how being sick makes you wonder this now." Unless patients ask you about your beliefs, support them to find their own answers to their religious questions. If the religiosity is assessed as harmful, then follow the guidelines in Chapter 6 for reconciling when patient and professional perspectives clash.

- Keep the conversation ball in the patient's court. Make your responses short, and then redirect the discourse to the patient.

- Focus on the core theme when responding to a patient's comments about religion. What is the main thought or feeling in what the patient said? What is the cutting edge element?

- Focus on the patient's experience, not the facts. For example, if a patient is describing how abandoned he feels because the church family no longer visits, then respond to the sense of abandonment or betrayal, rather than, "So which church did you attend?"

- Focus on the present. For example, how does the patient's religiosity influence the present? Or how will current religious experience affect the future? It is easy to avoid difficult topics like religious distress and doubts by focusing on the past or future; perhaps we hope for a glimmer of painlessness there. By focusing on the present experience, however, we support healing of such religion-related pain.

- Note a patient's use of religious terms and incorporate those (rather than yours). For example, if a person uses the term "God," do not use "Jesus" or "Higher Power." If a patient refers to her "faith community," do not assume that means church or synagogue or mosque and use such language. Using particularly charged words or phrases such as sin, repentance, salvation, born again, and so forth would not be wise unless the patient has already used such language. Again, you are following patient cues and responding to the patient's themes, not yours.

- Talk heart to heart or head to head (Carkhuff, 1969). While the above guidelines are likely review for you, this point may not be, and it is extremely helpful for conversations about such private topics as religiosity. This guideline informs which skill you use. That is, if a patient is speaking from the "head" (e.g., telling a story, talking about ideas, facts), then give a head response (i.e., restatement, open question). If the patient is speaking from close to the "heart" (e.g., describing feelings deep within, soul searching), then respond to the heart with a reflection of feelings. Often you will recognize speech from the heart because of the overt physical indicators that may accompany it, such as tears, guttural voice, or a big sigh. A patient who is talking from his head may be turned off by a nurse who responds with a reflection addressing the heart (feelings). Conversely, a patient who shares intimately from her heart about suffering will likely be disappointed and unaided by a nurse who asks her yet another fact-finding question.

Observing these guidelines will not only help you to remain therapeutic while talking with a patient about religion but will also facilitate ethical practice.

Skills for Communication About Religiosity

The skills most appropriate for supporting a patient to explore religiosity are those of making restatements, open questions, and empathy that names feelings. Although these skills are taught in every basic nursing training program, my experience has found that they are skills that remain undeveloped for most nurses. Therefore, a summary of these verbal communication skills with an eye to religious discourse follows.

Restatements

Restatements entail creating a condensed version of what a patient has said. The restatement should be not only shorter, but also clearer and more concrete. Restatements are helpful when the patient is having difficulty focusing their thoughts and they need help to hear what they are saying. The purpose of restatements is to clarify or focus the patient's thoughts (not feelings). Restatements can summarize or paraphrase the present or previous encounters (Hill, 2009). When creating a restatement:

- Consider what the most important theme is in what the patient is saying. Noting the nonverbal expressions, what aspect of the patient's narrative is given time and energy, as well as questions, conflicts, or unresolved issues the patient raises will help you to determine what is the most important theme.

- Remember you really do not know the patient's perspective. So be tentative with your words, tone of voice, and facial expression. Let patients feel comfortable correcting your observations as necessary. Phrases you can use include, "It seems as though . . . ," "I wonder if . . . ," "Maybe . . . ," or "Perhaps . . . ."

- Keep it short. A sentence is good (Egan, 2002; Hill, 2009; Taylor, 2007a).

Open questions
Open questions allow a patient to clarify and explore thoughts or feelings; they help the patient to consider "what's going on?" Nurses, however, are sometimes guilty of asking too many questions. Grilling a patient with questions can be an indicator of discomfort or need to control the conversation. When asking an open question, some points to remember are:

- Ask no more than two open questions in a row (Carkhuff, 1969). If the urge strikes, then rephrase your question into a restatement or reflection. For example, instead of asking "What kinds of answers does your religion offer for your question of 'why me'?" you can simply observe, "The 'why me?' question is really troubling you now." By remaining silently present, you allow the patient to respond. You can also avoid quizzing by asking a question indirectly. For example, ask "I wonder how your beliefs might begin to answer your question" instead of "How do your religious beliefs answer your question?"

- Ask about how's and what's. Avoid asking "why" questions, as they are threatening. For example, consider how assaultive it would be to be asked, "Why do you believe that?" instead of, "What helps you to believe this way?" Likewise, questions where an answer is implied are condescending (e.g., "You don't really believe that, do you?").

- Allow a patient to refuse to answer a question. A patient may not want to venture into the arena to which your question leads or at least not with you. Respect the patient's choice. You may respond with a restatement about what you are observing and offer a way you can care, if it is appropriate. For example, "I'm sensing that you don't feel like talking right now. Know that I care [pause, and move on]." (Egan, 2002; Hill, 2009; Taylor, 2007a).

Ultimately, you use open questions when you intuit they will be therapeutic, and helpful to the patient.

Reflecting feelings
"Feelings often provide a powerful window to the Holy" (Fischer, 2006). Reflecting feelings entails restating what feelings a patient has expressed verbally or nonverbally (Taylor, 2007a). Whereas it usually takes several words or phrases to describe a thought, it can take only one word to describe a feeling. Because we humans typically learn to minimize or hide our true feelings, having someone name them brings understanding and emotional release—healing. As the guidelines above stated, when a patient is speaking about their religion from the heart, then an empathic reflection is appropriate. The following suggestions will help you to formulate a reflection of feelings—a difficult skill to develop:

- Consider both the type of feeling experienced and the intensity of that feeling. A very simplified (yet easy to remember) categorization of feelings include bad, mad, sad, and glad. To illustrate how types of feelings can vary in intensity, think about the variations in sadness. To feel sad a little bit may mean feeling wistful, disappointed, or "a bit blue." More intense sad feelings include feeling mournful or being stricken with grief. Although you will do your best to name the correct type and intensity of feeling, know that you are guessing.

- Therefore, it is important to state your reflection in a tentative manner. This allows the patient to correct you—and contribute to the process of gaining greater appreciation for what the inner experience is.

- Although the basic formula for reflecting feelings is "you feel X because (or when) Y," this will probably sound unnatural and formulaic. Other ways to name another's feelings include encapsulating the feeling in a word, phrase, experiential statement, or behavioral statement. If, for example, a patient was tearfully describing how "God seems a million light-years away from me here," feeling reflective responses might include: "Feeling alone (or disconnected, or abandoned)?" (feeling in a word); "Sort of feel hung out to dry" (feeling in a phrase, such as a metaphor); "Feels like God doesn't care maybe" (feeling of abandonment or rejection implied in an experiential statement); "Might make you feel like giving up on God" (feeling is implied by saying what action the patient might feel like taking) (Egan, 2002; Hill, 2009; Taylor, 2007a).

These guidelines and skills for talking therapeutically about any topic, including religion, should steer nurse–patient discourse.

CONVERSATION ABOUT RELIGIOSITY: AVOIDING HARM

When a patient raises a sensitive topic such as religion, this topic can be too discomforting for the nurse who may then run away or shut up the patient. One way some religious nurses may try to comfort is by offering religious comments intended to give hope but, in reality, can be hurtful or cause harm. This section describes some of the ways this happens.

When Religious Conversation Gets Too Heavy: Escape Techniques

If a nurse is not religious, a religious patient's comments about religion may irritate, bemuse, or mystify a nurse, making him or her uncomfortable with the topic. Likewise, for even the religious nurse, a patient's expressions of religious struggle, doubt, betrayal, and so forth, can be very disturbing and difficult to hear. These are unfixables; nurses prefer fixables. Therefore, the tendency in such situations is for the nurse to silence or leave the patient. This can be done unknowingly and under the illusion of self-protection. Common escape techniques used include:

- Tending to tasks, doing the doable. Running away from a difficult conversation is "legitimized" when it is for a good reason like obtaining medication—or so a nurse may tell herself. For the patient who may be feeling desperate and has summoned much courage to broach the topic with the nurse, however, such a nurse response is one of avoidance and potentially hurts the therapeutic relationship.

- Changing the topic. This can be accomplished by going off on a tangent or introducing another subject that you know is important to the patient.

- Minimizing the intensity of the pain. For a rude example, "Oh, it couldn't be that bad!" More commonly, however, you may hear an interjection of positivity to minimize pain, such as "Look at all you still have to be thankful for." Often humor is used to minimize the perception of spiritual pain. While these techniques may be therapeutic after the pain has been named and opportunity for exploration has been given, it is not therapeutic if it is used to escape the pain.

- Responding with a superficial answer. Many of the religiously oriented struggles patients have are ultimately mysteries. In our finite humanness that loves control and certainty, it is difficult to live with such struggle.

- Providing a positive spin. For example, "Although your pain here on earth is hard to live with, remember that it is insignificant compared to the painlessness you'll have in eternal life." A nurse's desperation to comfort self and patient drives the need to inject a positive angle in response to religious distress. Again, while it may be therapeutic to make such a statement (if it has been assessed that such a statement is congruent with the patient's beliefs), it is unlikely to be helpful if used as a quick escape.

- Praying. As with providing a pat answer or positive spin, "using" prayer can be an effective means for bringing premature closure to discomforting religious discourse. Indeed, some patients have learned that asking for prayer is a good way to get rid of clergy or clinicians who are no longer welcome.

Using such techniques, of course, challenges the trust the patient may have in the nurse and remove an opportunity for truly holistic healing to occur. While it may be that a nurse does not have the skills or time for addressing distressing religious issues, it is best in such circumstances to name the concern and make a referral or negotiate a later time for such discourse rather than to avoid and devalue the issue. For example, "I'm sensing you're really hurting deep down about not being at peace with God; would it be okay if I ask an expert at dealing with these sorts of concerns to come and talk with you?"

Hurtful Religious Statements

It is also possible for a religious nurse comforting a distressed patient with religious admonitions to instead cause hurt or harm. Consider the following examples identified by Taylor (2002):

- "Just pray about it." For patients experiencing God as distant during prayer or unable to pray in the ways they are used to, this admonition may bring a sense of guilt or awareness of frustration. Instead, the patient would likely benefit from expanded ways of thinking about what prayer is and how to pray when sick (Taylor, 2003).

- "Just leave it in the Lord's hands." If this statement is interpreted as, "Be passive, disengage," it may undermine coping. Research on the psychology of religious coping indicates that passive religious coping is associated with poorer adaptation than an active or collaborative religious coping that occurs when a patient collaborates with the divine to cope with illness issues (Ano & Vasconcelles, 2005; Pargament, Koenig, & Perez, 2000). Thus, it is possible that passive, ineffective coping is encouraged by such a statement.

- "God doesn't give you more than you can bear" or "God is testing you; stand strong." The patient may feel that the degree of suffering *is* more than he or she can bear. Comments such as this may convey an unsettling perspective of a sinister deity.

- "It must be God's will" or "It's part of God's plan." Statements like this often represent an attempt to avoid complex subjects.

- "Don't let the devil get the best of you." Such a statement infers a negative religious coping framing, an approach found by psychological research to be maladaptive (Ano & Vasconcelles, 2005; Pargament, Koenig, & Perez, 2000). Indeed, comments that introduce ideas of punishment, abandonment, or direct evil effects in the context of illness are likely psychologically and spiritually harmful.

These statements illustrate how the religious perspectives and maturity of a nurse can be unveiled at the bedside. Although a nurse who offers such responses to a patient may have the sincerest of intentions, they nevertheless display religious insensitivity. Indeed, openness toward the continued mysteries (unanswerable questions) that all world religions embrace is a healthful stance for nurses.

When Patients Ask Nurses About Their Religion: Helpful Self-Disclosure

Sometimes it is appropriate to self-disclose personal beliefs. It should be done, however, only for therapeutic purposes while following patient cues. Unethical proselytizing never comes from patient need and always from a nurse's need.

Patients ask nurses about their religiosity for various reasons (Taylor, 2002). The patient may simply be curious or want to build a bridge of friendship to the nurse by inquiring about the nurse's personal life. The patient may also be checking to see if it is safe to talk about religion with the nurse, looking for religious information and perceives the nurse as one source, or intuit that this technique is a good one for getting off track from uncomfortable dialog. Whatever the reason, a patient's transference is revealed in their querying about your religion (Tillman, 1998). Thus, understanding why a patient inquires about a nurse's religiosity should inform that nurse's response.

The following guidance (Taylor, 2007a) on religious self-disclosure can promote therapeutic conversation and prevent unethical proselytization:

- Assess. The nurse must inwardly ask, "Whose needs am I meeting by sharing my personal beliefs?" Also, try to determine why the patient is inquiring about your religion. For example, "I'm happy to share about what I believe, but I'm wondering what brings you to ask?"

- Make the self-disclosure brief and focused so as to meet the patient's need (e.g., for information, for relationship, for safety).

- Conclude by placing the ball in the patient's court. For example, "I've just shared my viewpoint; I wonder what yours is?"

Keep in mind the risks of self-disclosure not only include unethical coercion of beliefs, but can also be a means for sidetracking from more painful core issues. Self-disclosure also creates the risk making yourself an exemplar for the patient.

Avoiding Harm From Incompetence

Religious conversations with patients can reveal very deep spiritual and emotional pain. What is the role of nurses with regard to such angst? Should nurses even encourage patients to express such pain? Can harm be done by leading a patient to express such pain when the nurse is incapable of addressing it? Nurse ethicist and theologian Fowler (in Pesut, Fowler, Reimer-Kirkham, Taylor, & Sawatzky, 2009) argued that, indeed, nurses can cause harm if treading into patient religious experience for which they are ill equipped and if it is not within the purview of nursing.

Fowler (Pesut et al., 2009) proposed there are layers of spirituality, akin to layers of an onion, where the outer layer of public spirituality covers successively intimate layers of spirituality. For instance, a patient's outer and most public spirituality is the territory where nurses talk about nonsensitive facts (e.g., "What church do you attend?"). Below that is a semipublic spirituality where religious facts are selectively disclosed (e.g., "I often pray for healing"). Going inward to deeper layers reveals spiritual struggles of which the patient is aware (e.g., "I'm beginning to think God doesn't care"), and then to deep inner struggles for which it is difficult to give voice (e.g., doubting the nature or existence of a God). Fowler posited that unless the nurse has received advanced training (e.g., chaplaincy, spiritual direction), the nurse is not prepared to venture into patient religiosity deeper than the outer two layers (i.e., public and semipublic religiosity). Thus, given nurses generally do not possess such training, it is imperative that nurses "stand on holy ground" with much caution, not advancing into to religious territory where they are not trained to enter.

Remembering their role as spiritual care generalists—not experts (Taylor, 2002)—nurses ought to work closely with experts whose role and training allow them closer to the "burning bush" (to continue the Mosaic analogy). Nurses can perform a pivotal role in facilitating referrals. Given that most institutions are poorly staffed with chaplains, it is nurses who can screen patients for expert care and make a referral to the appropriate expert (e.g., chaplain, clergy, spiritual director, or mental health specialist appreciative of the impact of religion on health).

MAKING SENSE OF PATIENTS' RELIGIOUS TALK

As every nurse learns, communicating involves not only sending verbal and nonverbal messages, but also receiving them. Whereas the previous sections of this chapter have focused on sending messages, this section will discuss how to make sense of messages you receive from the patient who is talking about religion.

Analyzing Religious Conversation

As you listen to patients talk about their religiosity, there are several angles to consider that can help you to make sense of what they say. Summarizing the chaplaincy and counseling literature in this regard, Taylor (2007a) listed the following suggestions:

- What patients say to you at first reflects not how well you asked a good question but how safe and respected the patient feels with you. Superficial religious clichés or tangential comments can indicate that a patient simply is not comfortable going deeper with you at the present time. Rapport and relationship, after all, is what patients want from a nurse who is offering spiritual care (Taylor, 2007b).

- Consider what sorts of incongruities exist. Are there any incongruities between affect, behavior, and communication (ABCs) shown by the patient? Does what the patient say about himself match what he wants to be? Do what the patient says and does match? Any incongruities you might observe suggest what areas the patient may benefit from exploring with you or an expert.

- Weigh how abstract or concrete is the patient's description of religiosity. Often those who speak abstractly or conceptually are distancing themselves from thoughts and feelings they fear. In contrast, when a patient uses concrete speech too much, it can indicate an anxiety about considering the more abstract meanings or implications of a belief. A healthy religiosity straddles the extremes of abstractness and concreteness.

• Reflect on how defensive or threatened the patient is by talk about religion. Just as nurses can avoid religion-related distress using the techniques listed above, so also can patients (e.g., changing the topic, letting the nurse do all the talking). A patient who is defensive may also become competitive (e.g., gives lots of scriptural quotes or facts to show their knowledge), or intellectualize their feelings. Such defensiveness is best counteracted by being present as a sojourner in life or by modeling comfort with talking about religious matters. As needed, divert to a less threatening topic or recommend a referral to a spiritual care expert.

• Keep in mind that crises expose the gaps in a patient's faith development. Healers allow patients to explore these gaps and grow through them. Faith development involves learning about beliefs and practices concretely as a child, then abstractly as cognitive development allows. It involves learning from parents, then differentiating from these spiritual beliefs and practices as one enters teenage and young adulthood, and creating a satisfying personal belief system as one becomes an adult. Adult spiritual development often involves phases of re-searching for satisfying beliefs and meaningful practices (Fowler, 1981).

• Keep in mind that religion offers a lens for interpreting life. When a person talks about religion, they are talking about their world.

• "Tell me what you find in the Bible, and I will tell you what you are," a friend of Freud's wrote (Dayringer, 1998). When patients tell you a religious story, they are telling you about themselves. How patients use and interpret their religious Scripture can be a diagnostic that informs a nurse about a patient's personality and beliefs.

• Think about how helpful is the patient's religiosity. Religious beliefs are helpful for patients to the degree that these beliefs foster emotional health, positive relationships, and hope (Griffith & Griffith, 2002). Unhelpful religion includes:

  • Undifferentiated or one-sided religiosity (when a narrow aspect of religion is pursued)

  • Fragmented religiosity (when behaviors are incongruent with beliefs)

  • Inflexible, rigid religiosity (which prevents one from considering various religious perspectives to interpret stressful circumstances)

  • Insecure attachments to the divine or faith community (Cole, Benore, & Pargament, 2004).

If unhelpful religiosity is observed, make a referral so that helpful religious coping skills can be enhanced. Respect, however, even unhealthy religiosity, as it would be cruel to unravel patients' unhealthy religiosity when it may be their only source of comfort.

Evaluating Effectiveness of Communication

Whether you have responded to a patient's religiosity with a restatement, question, feeling reflection, or self-disclosure, you will want to note whether your response to their expressed religious concern was therapeutic. You can do so by gauging the patient's response. That is, did what you say stimulate the patient to continue exploration or to gain insight about their religious experience? Did it encourage them to continue to reflect on their issue? Did it bring a sense of relief that the distress was named or given voice? Indicators of effectiveness not only include having the patient continue to grapple with an issue, but also sighing with "Yes, that's it" or a nonverbal indicator of becoming more aware of inner experience.

PUTTING IT ALL TOGETHER

We began by asking how a nurse should respond to a religious patient who pushes her buttons or how a religious nurse might discuss helpful religious coping. Instead of answering these questions directly, this chapter has presented principles and guidelines that can help nurses to respond to these and other scenarios involving religious discourse. These guidelines remind nurses of the importance of patient-centered communication—even (or especially) when talking about religion. Instead of being unsettled by a patient's religious talk, these guidelines give a nurse appreciation for the deeper meanings inherent in such discourse and skills for responding in a way that will help patients to explore how their religiosity impacts their well-being (e.g., making a restatement or asking an open question that appreciates the theme at the core of the patient's talk). Likewise, the nurse who wants to share personally helpful religiosity is given suggestions for when and how to make a patient-centered, therapeutic self-disclosure. Ultimately, nurse–patient conversations about religion must reflect the patient's health-related need, not the nurse's need.

PRIMARY PRACTICE POINTS

- A nurse should talk about religion only if the patient introduces it or if it is necessary for reasons related to nursing and health care.

- If the goal for the nurse–patient discourse about religion is not to assess, then it is to support the patient in exploring (so as to gain insight and resolve distress) how their religious experience has an impact on health.

- Nurse responses to patient expression of religiosity must be nonauthoritarian and patient-centered; therapeutic responses will match whether the patient speaks from the "head" or the "heart."

- Communication skills most appropriate for such discourse include restatements, open questions, and empathic reflections of feelings. Self-disclosures of personal religiosity should occur only after it has been determined to be therapeutic.

- Nurses can do harm when escaping religion-related distress by offering superficial answers, imposing a positive spin, minimizing, or in other ways avoiding the pain.

- Nurses can also inadvertently cause harm by delving into deep religious pain for which they are untrained or unable to address. It is important for nurses to appreciate their valuable role as spiritual care generalists and make referrals to specialists when it is needed.

- Some questions that can help nurses to make sense of what religious patients are saying include: How helpful is religion in this patient's life? (Is it integrating or dis-integrating?) How does religion offer an interpretive lens for life for this patient? Are there incongruities or defensiveness when religious experience is described?

REFERENCES

Ano, G., & Vasconcelles, E. (2005). Religious coping and psychological adjustment to stress: A meta-analysis. *Journal of Clinical Psychology, 61*, 461–480.

Baranowsky, A. B. (2002). The silencing response in clinical practice: On the road to dialogue. In C. R. Figley (Ed.), *Treating compassion fatigue* (Chapter 8). New York, NY: Brunner-Routledge.

Burleson, B. R. (2003). Emotional support skills. In J. O. Greene & B. R. Burleson (Eds.), *Handbook of communication and social interaction skills*. Mahwah, NJ: Lawrence Erlbaum Associates.

Carkhuff, R. R. (1969). *Helping and human relations: A primer for lay and professional helpers*. Volume 1. Selection and training. New York, NY: Holt, Rinehart, & Winston.

Cole, B., Benore, E., & Pargament, K. (2004). Spirituality and coping with trauma. In S. Sirajjakool & H. Lamberton (Eds.), *Spirituality, health, & wholeness: An introductory guide for health care professionals* (pp. 49–76). New York, NY: Haworth Press.

Dayringer, R. (1998). *The heart of pastoral counseling: Healing through relationship*. (Rev. ed.). New York, NY: Haworth Pastoral Press.

Egan, G. (2002). *The skilled helper: A problem-management and opportunity-development approach to helping* (7th ed.). Pacific Grove, CA: Brooks/Cole.

Fischer, K. (2006). Working with the emotions in spiritual direction: Seven guiding principles. *Presence: An International Journal of Spiritual Direction, 12*(3), 26–35.

Fowler, J. W. (1981). *Stages of faith development: The psychology of human development and the quest for meaning*. San Francisco, CA: Harper & Row.

Griffith, J. L., & Griffith, M. E. (2002). *Encountering the sacred in psychotherapy*. New York, NY: Guilford.

Hill, C. E. (2009). *Helping skills: Facilitating exploration, insight, and action* (3rd ed.). Washington, DC: American Psychological Association.

Pargament, K., Koenig, H., & Perez, L. (2000). The many methods of religious coping: Development and validation of the RCOPE. *Journal of Clinical Psychology, 56,* 519–543.

Pesut, B., Fowler, M., Reimer-Kirkham, S., Taylor, E. J., & Sawatzky, R. (2009). Particularizing spirituality in points of tension: Enriching the discourse. *Nursing Inquiry, 16*(4), 337–346.

Taylor, E. J. (2002). *Spiritual care: Nursing theory, research, and practice.* Upper Saddle River, NJ: Prentice Hall.

Taylor, E. J. (2003). Prayer's clinical issues and implications. *Holistic Nursing Practice, 17,* 179–188.

Taylor, E. J. (2007a). *What do I say? Talking with patients about spirituality.* Philadelphia, PA: Templeton.

Taylor, E. J. (2007b). Client perspectives about nurse requisites for spiritual caregiving. *Applied Nursing Research, 20*(1), 44–46.

Tillman, J. G. (1998). Psychodynamic psychotherapy, religious beliefs, and self-disclosure. *American Journal of Psychotherapy Practice and Research, 52,* 273–286.

Assessing Religiosity

Elizabeth Johnston Taylor, PhD, RN

A n oncology nurse wrote about this episode of religious care:

> My patient was in end stage of his cancer. His vital signs were awful, he was mottled, his level of consciousness was fluctuating. He was very restless and anxious. As soon as he appeared to be restful, his eyes would pop open and he'd again begin to struggle. His wife and I assured him of our love and support. I asked him if he was afraid to die. He answered affirmatively. I asked him what his religion was. His wife responded for him stating he was Protestant. I then reviewed Christian belief in afterlife with him and provided the video "Life after Life" by Dr. Moody. The patient became calm and died shortly afterwards.

In this vignette, although we may challenge why the nurse was compelled to assure the patient of her love and support, we do see the effects of a cursory religious assessment. We also see, however, the potential for harm from a nurse using an "intervention" describing psychological research into near-death experiences to prove there is an immediate afterlife for a patient who could have been an adherent of a Protestant tradition with differing theology. For example, a Seventh-Day Adventist believes death is like sleep, with the Second Advent of Jesus bringing resurrection of the dead from the dust to which they went at death. Other conservative Christians may be leery about "new age" depictions of near-death experiences portrayed in this video. So for varying reasons, some patients—even though assessed as Protestant—could be quite discomforted by watching such a video. Indeed, this nurse wrote that she reviewed Christian beliefs about life after death with the patient. Whose beliefs were shared? Was it appropriate for this nurse to function as a purveyor of theology? Although religious affiliation was assessed, did this nurse also assess for how the patient desired support?

Asking anybody about his or her religion can be really tough. It can create awkwardness and embarrassment, for both the person asking and the one answering the query. Given the traditional taboos against discussing politics, sex, and religion in social conversations, such an assessment could even offend. This chapter, therefore, will not only discuss various aspects of assessing religion, but also explore techniques for improving a clinician's comfort with asking patients questions about religiosity.

WHY ASSESS RELIGIOSITY?

A few thoughtful physicians and ethicists raise the question of whether it is appropriate to assess religiosity given the high risk it creates for moving clinician from the role of health care provider to that of spiritual advisor (Cohen et al., 2001; Post, Puchalski, & Larson, 2000). Cohen and colleagues in the Anglican Working Group on Bioethics sum the issue up:

> The real issue is not whether religions and spiritual commitments improve patients' health but rather whether physician [or nurse] inquiries into such commitments honor patients as persons. What justifies such inquiries is the recognition of patients as whole and integrated persons with the right and responsibility to govern their medical [and health] care in accord with the fundamental beliefs by which they order their lives. (p. 32)

Understanding the religious beliefs that are influencing a patient's decision regarding whether to pursue a life-extending treatment, for example, can help a nurse to assist the patient to make an embraceable, congruent choice. Knowing the specifics of a religious practice with health implications will allow a nurse to offer pertinent information and aid. Thus, approaches to learning about patient religiosity vis-à-vis health are needed.

ASSESSING SPIRITUALITY OR RELIGIOSITY?

Religiosity is always considered an aspect of spiritual assessment in nursing literature on the topic. In reality, however, the two concepts are often confused. Most recommendations regarding spiritual assessment advise at least a two-stepped approach (Massey, Fitchett, & Roberts, 2004; Puchalski et al., 2009; Taylor, 2010). First, a screening assessment is needed to determine superficially if there are any spiritual or religious beliefs and practices that are important to the patient and what, if anything, the patient would want from the health care provider/s as far as spiritual or religious support. Such a screening will presumably determine if there even is a spiritual reality for the patient (Pesut, Fowler, Reimer-Kirkham, Taylor, & Sawatzky, 2009). Once it is established that there are spiritual or religious concerns or beliefs or practices that are important to the patient, the clinician is advised to conduct a more in-depth interview. Taylor (2002) suggests that this more in-depth spiritual assessment explore only the specific concern raised during the screening. Thus, an assessment of religiosity would follow an initial spirituality screening that ascertains religiosity does have an impact on a patient's health or response to a health-related transition.

WHEN SHOULD RELIGIOSITY BE ASSESSED?

If indeed a spiritual screening has identified that the patient has religious beliefs or practices, does that mean an assessment of religiosity should be started? Not necessarily. Hodge (2006) proposed several criteria for whether a clinician should commence a more in-depth spiritual assessment. These criteria apply especially to the assessment of religiosity. Framing the criteria as questions, they include:

- *Is religion relevant or important to the patient?* Although a patient may self-identify as of a particular religious tradition, that religion may not be important to him or her. One may have a sense of belonging to the tradition, but not believe in it (e.g., atheistic Jew). While for many, such nominal religiosity will still have its subtle influences (and in times of crises become an important issue), it is possible that it is not relevant enough to warrant further assessment.

- *Does the patient give consent to further assessment of religiosity?* Does the patient want you to probe more deeply? Often, rather religious persons are quite comfortable talking about their religiosity with anyone. Because they are steeped in their religion, they have the language and experience with which to discuss religious experience. For some, however, religious matters remain very intimate and only open for discussion with safe persons (e.g., nurses who are similarly minded or established as empathic and respectful). The Western ethical principle of respect for the autonomy of persons dictates that nurses get some sense of approval from a patient when delving into such a topic. However, for patients from collectivist cultures (e.g., Asian), this consent may need to come from family members involved in the health care. Either way, a simple question such as "Would you like to talk about how your [your loved one's] religious beliefs or practices might influence the way you [he or she] want/s to be cared for?" should suffice (Dehaven, 2001).

- *Are you competent to conduct the assessment of religiosity?* Not only does the nurse need to be knowledgeable about aspects of religiosity and how to assess these, but also culturally and psychologically safe for the patient. That is, the nurse who is culturally safe is unthreatened by learning about another's religion. This nurse is able to be nonjudgmental, respectful, and sensitive as a listener and interviewer. Competence also requires a nurse to work at self-awareness about religion. This nurse will not counter transfer his or her preestablished thinking about religion into the assessment process.

- *Is information about the patient's religiosity relevant to health?* The nurse should limit an assessment of religion to aspects that are pertinent to health. If a screening shows a patient to be religious, then a follow-up for a new patient might be "In what ways do you think I might need to know more about your religious beliefs or practices?" or "How does your religion have an impact on the way you take care of your health?" If you are caring for a patient facing a particular circumstance, then you can tailor the follow-up to suit that circumstance. For example, "As you are trying to decide which treatment option to take, tell me how—if at all—your religious beliefs come in to play." For assessment purposes, to venture beyond religiosity vis-à-vis health is not within the role of nursing, or as Johnson and Nielsen (1998) propose, ask: "Does maximal therapeutic gain hinge on a focal assessment of the nature of religious belief and expression?" (p. 111). A nurse's curiosity or agenda to proselytize are never good reasons to initiate any assessment of religion.

These criteria for whether to move beyond a screening to a more focused, in-depth assessment establish that there are conditions for when an assessment of religiosity is not warranted or wanted. Even when a nurse assesses that religion is salient in the life of a patient but the patient does not consent to further assessment, it is helpful to remember that an assessment that is coerced is unlikely to yield either accurate or in-depth information. In such a situation, the nurse can make a referral or work to develop better rapport with the patient.

WHO SHOULD ASSESS RELIGIOSITY?

Should every nurse be skilled at assessing patient religiosity? If not, what factors should determine who ought to do it? Should the level of assessment reflect the skill and preparation of the nurse?

Although The Joint Commission (2005) allows accredited institutions to choose who completes the required spiritual assessment, most health care organizations relegate the responsibility to nurses. Hospitals typically then include one to three questions about spirituality and religion in a nursing intake assessment form. Often, admission clerks ask patients if there is a religion with which they identify. While such processes ascertain religious affiliation, they typically do not learn the nature of that affiliation, never mind more pertinent information about what aspects of that religion the patient perceives as important to health.

A model for determining who should assess religiosity is offered by Marsha Fowler (Pesut et al., 2009), a nurse ethicist and spiritual care scholar. This model posits that the level of assessment should reflect the skill and preparation of the nurse. Because skills will vary among nurses given their varied formal and informal preparation in religious assessment, the expectation for what level of assessment they perform should vary. Not only does the nurse skill vary, but the nature or complexity of the patient's religious experience varies. Fowler's model asserts that patient religiosity is like an onion with layers of increasing depth:

- The outermost layer is that of public religiosity, factual information that can be disclosed to strangers. For example, "Yes, I'm Catholic, I went to parochial schools; no, I don't attend church any longer."

- Underneath that layer, there is another that is semipublic. That is, a layer of information that is still largely factual that is disclosed to more specific persons, such as closer acquaintances, perhaps coworkers: "No, I don't go to church any longer because. . . ."

- Beneath that is a third layer that becomes more intimate as individuals wrestle with spiritual or religious concerns within their awareness. This layer may or may not be shared with family, but is commonly shared with a specific, intimate, and caring friend. It is not unusual here for persons to seek pastoral counseling from trusted faith community leaders.

- Peeling away that layer, there is the fourth layer of troubling feelings, guilt, or concerns that the person often cannot articulate precisely. This, too, is a layer for a trusted religious leader (spiritual advisor); one that requires deeper exploration to crystallize the issues and help them emerge into the person's awareness.

- Beneath that layer is a layer where the darknesses of spiritual life are encountered. These must be dealt with either because circumstances have made them visible or because the person is seeking spiritual growth and is ready to wrestle with them. This layer is the purview of a trained spiritual director.

Fowler asserts that there are more layers, including the most inward core where no person can go unless God takes them there. But for our discussion, it is vital to appreciate that these "layers" involve progressive levels of depth, ineffability, and intimacy.

The public and semipublic layers are open to all nurses and are part of expected data collection: religious affiliation, religious practices, and the like. The third layer enters into particulars: what one's tradition believes about health; responsibility for health or caregiving; how one's tradition views mental illness, suffering, or end of life treatment; and the extent to which the patient agrees or disagrees. This layer of spiritual assessment can be that of nursing but requires that the nurse have a solid understanding of religious traditions to know if the patient is consistent with the formal positions of that tradition and to assist the patient in his or her incorporation of that tradition.

After the first two layers, there is a need for education in religion and spirituality that exceeds that which is customarily provided in nursing education. Nurses formally prepared in spiritual care, that is, those whose primary clinical expertise and specialized preparation is in spiritual care, do move in to the third layer. However, they do so only in relation to nursing's domain of health, illness, trauma, and not for the purpose of spiritual direction or formation. These purposes are for those dedicated to full time spiritual care. Spiritual pain resides beneath the layers that unspecialized nurses should not enter. At times, nurses enter unaware, or even by painful invitation of the suffering patient, but to do so is to incur risk both for themselves and for the patient.

Although nurses play an integral role in assessing religiosity, it is important to remember that spiritual and religious assessments are ideally completed by various members of a health care team (Timmins & Kelly, 2008). A spiritual care expert and a mental health professional, for example, can provide more depth to an assessment.

HOW CAN RELIGIOSITY BE ASSESSED?

The assessment of religiosity can be done with intake questionnaires or clinical interviews using a variety of strategies. While intake questionnaires are befitting of screening and assessment of public or semiprivate religiosity, the clinical interview strategies offer means for more in-depth assessment. Either approach may be complemented by use of standardized assessment measures.

Intake Questions for Screening Patients

Given the purpose to screen for religiosity and religious issues, intake questions that "cut to the chase" may be most useful. Many health care professionals have offered examples of spiritual screening questions that include reference to religiosity (Taylor, 2010). These include

- I was wondering if spirituality or religion is important to you? Or, How important is spirituality or religion to you? Or, Would you describe yourself—in the broadest sense of the term—as a believing or religious person?

- Is your religion (or faith) helpful to you in handling your illness? Or, Is faith/religion important to you in this illness/in your life? Or, Are there certain spiritual beliefs and practices that you find particularly helpful in dealing with problems?

- Are there aspects of your religion you would like me to keep in mind as I care for you?

Puchalski & Romer's (2000) mnemonic "FICA" allows a clinician to remember facets of religiosity for assessment. This popular approach is as follows: F (does the patient have a faith or beliefs?), I (what is the importance or influence of religion?), C (for community—is the patient a part of a religious community?), and A (for address—how does the patient want religious issues addressed by the health care provider/s?). Although several such mnemonics (Taylor, 2010) exist for spiritual assessment, FICA is likely the most widely cited and easily used; it is also the tool most focused specifically on religiosity.

Exhibit 3.1 offers an example of a spiritual screening assessment that includes religiosity that would work well in an admission interview. Such a screening will identify patients who are religious, those who will benefit from further religious assessment, and how the health care team can support patient religiosity.

EXHIBIT 3.1
Admission Spiritual Screening That Includes Religiosity

How important is spirituality, faith, or religion
to you?*

___ Not applicable
___ Not at all
___ Somewhat
___ A lot

*An alternative question to
consider is:

Which would best describe
yourself?

___ Neither religious nor spiritual
___ Spiritual, but not religious
___ Religious, but not spiritual
___ Both religious and spiritual

Are there aspects of your religion or spirituality you would like us to keep in
mind as we care for you?

___ Prayer/meditation

___ Being involved with my faith community

___ Inspirational books/music/media

___ Diet: please explain _____

___ Other practices or religious observances:

___ Beliefs pertinent to health care: please describe:

Please list any religious affiliation/s:

Would you like us to contact someone from whom you would want spiritual or
religious support?

___ No
___ Yes: Please list contact information:

Name:

Title/role:

Telephone:

Other necessary information:
Additional comments:

Clinical Interviews for Assessing Religious Patients

Once it is known that religion—to some degree—influences the patient's response to health challenges, the nurse can determine if a more in-depth assessment of religiosity is appropriate. That is, is information about the patient's religion pertinent to the health care you want to deliver? Assuming you believe you are competent to assess religiosity, then you will want to obtain the patient's permission. You can introduce the assessment in a way that explains why you are doing it and gain the patient's consent. For example:

- I noticed on the admissions' assessment that you are a person of faith. For many people, faith gives a way of thinking and coping with health problems. How is it for you?

- Your health care team is about to discuss your treatment options. We know that often patients have religious beliefs that affect the way they make decisions. Do you mind telling me more about how your beliefs might affect the way you are dealing with your illness?

Of course, respectful verbal and nonverbal nurse responses are vital. Such assessing often brings to the fore references to religious concerns, doubts, struggles, hurts.

Several clinicians offer clinical interview guides for spiritual and religious assessment (Taylor, 2010), which cover a gamut of facets of religiosity. While some are simply listings of open questions covering various aspects of religiosity (Nelson-Becker, Nakashim, & Canda, 2007; Ortiz & Langer, 2002), others are assessment forms allowing tick box (Hay, 1989) or scaled responses (Mohr, Gillieron, Borras, Brandt, & Huguelet, 2007).

Other approaches to a clinical interview exist. Hodge (2005) identified several creative approaches to collecting information about client spirituality that are just as easily used to assess religiosity. As a social worker, Hodge is well aware that some patients are not verbal or are not comfortable expressing their spirituality or religiosity in words. Thus, he explained more visual ways for a patient to describe their spiritual experiences. Two of these methods for assessment most likely to be useful for nurses include:

- Spiritual lifemaps, or a pictoral depiction of where the patient has been spiritually, where the patient is presently, and where the patient expects to go. It can be a simple pencil drawing on a large piece of paper; words and illustrations can be used to convey the spiritual story—the spiritual highs and lows, blessings and burdens, and so forth.

- Spiritual ecomaps, rather than focusing on past spiritual influences, direct the patient to consider present spiritual experience. In particular, the patient can diagram (with self portrayed in the center) the relationship with God or transcendent other/value, rituals, faith community, and encounters with other spiritual entities.

Other strategies include having clients draw a spiritual timeline that includes significant books, experiences, events, and so forth. Another unusual approach involves sentence completion. For example, a client may fill in the blank of sentences like "My relation to God . . ." or "What I would really like to be . . ." or "When I feel overwhelmed. . . ." Having verbally oriented assessment strategies as well as these nonverbal methods provides clinicians with a "toolbox" for assessing spirituality, allowing the clinician to choose an approach that fits the patient's personality, circumstances, and purpose for assessment.

Standardized Assessment Measures

While some argue for flexible, personable approaches to assessing religiosity or spirituality that are not reductionistic (McSherry & Ross, 2002; O'Connor et al., 2005), others advocate for use of structured and standardized instruments for ease of documentation and evaluation (Puchalski et al., 2009). Criteria for selecting a standardized tool to measure religiosity of a patient include:

• Is there established validity for the tool, especially in a short version?

• Is the tool reliable, especially for the patient population you serve?

• Is the tool culturally sensitive? (e.g., appropriate for the diverse religiosity you see?)

• Is the tool brief, easy to complete in only a few minutes?

• Is the tool easily understood, with simple language?

Most importantly, perhaps, is the question of whether the instrument measures something that the health care team (or patient) would benefit from measuring.

Standardized measures of religiosity with potential for clinical use include the following: the Koenig, Patterson, and Meador 5-item Duke University Religion Index that measures frequency of organizational religious activities as well as personal religious spirituality (Hill & Hood, 1999); the 14-item Brief RCOPE, which measures use of positive and negative religious coping (Pargament, Feuille, & Burdzy, 2011); and Gorsuch and McPherson's 14-item Religious Orientation Scale-Revised, which differentiates religiosity as being primarily intrinsically and extrinsically motivated (Hill & Hood).

How Can Religiosity Be Assessed Without Embarrassment?

One reason nurses fail to assess spirituality and religiosity is because they think such questions are intrusive (Swift, Calcuttawalla, & Elliot, 2007). Indeed, one's religiosity can be an extremely private matter, especially in some cultures. Some approaches that will minimize embarrassment for both the patient and nurse include:

• *Gain awareness of personal prejudicial attitudes for and against religions.* This will help the nurse to not project personal attitudes into the assessment process. Unless checked, such projections will be sensed by the patient and anger or silence them. When exploring another's religion, it is paramount that one work to "decolonize" the assessment of the "religious other" (Louw, 1999).

- *Create rapport and trust.* Show that you genuinely care for, honor, and respect the patient. You can only do this, however, if you have a genuine interest in exploring (versus renovating) the patient's religiosity (Johnson & Nielsen, 1998). In a small qualitative study (*N*=10), Ellis and Campbell (2004) found that these were patients' prerequisites for discussions about spiritual issues. Similarly, Taylor (2007) found that patients and family carers ranked a warm and trusting relationship as more important requisites to spiritual care than a shared religious perspective or even the nurse having training in spiritual care. Understanding at least a little about the social customs of the patient's religion will help you to not make a faux paus during assessment and cause the patient to clam up (Blass, 2007).

- *Introduce the assessment of religiosity with rationale.* Knowing how sharing more about their religiosity will help them will likely lower patient defenses.

- *Preferably, introduce the assessment when the patient is alone.* Not only can this lower the patient's discomfort, it will also support more forthright responses.

- *When patients express religious doubts, questions, and hurts, legitimize it.* Let them know that it is acceptable—even healing, to express such distress (Taylor, 2007). Assessment of religion actually begins a process of care. Having the opportunity and safety to express such concerns allows the patient to hear the self who is speaking; in that hearing comes awareness and inner growth.

- *Use the language the patient uses for key religious concepts.* For example, if a patient refers to wanting to "get right with their Maker," do not assume that their Maker is labeled God or that getting right means "repenting from sin."

Informal and Indirect Approaches

A nurse whose ears, eyes, and heart are continually receptive to patient messages will likely learn much about the religious patient's beliefs and practices without formally asking questions about religion. In clinical "chatter" about what the patient did over the weekend or during recent holidays (which often have religious underpinnings), or during a family member's rite of passage (rituals which often contain religious elements), the nurse can often get glimpses of the patient's religiosity. Likewise, observing religious jewelry, dress, dietary preferences, home décor, and greetings cards can give clues as to the patient's religiosity.

WHAT ASPECTS OF RELIGIOSITY SHOULD BE ASSESSED?

It is vital to reiterate that an in-depth or comprehensive assessment of every aspect of a patient's religiosity is inappropriate, unethical, and unnecessary for the nurse to complete. Except for nurses with advanced training in spiritual direction or pastoral care, nurses do not possess either adequate training about how to complete an in-depth assessment of religiosity or the skill to respond to expressions of complex religious issues that arise during an assessment and require immediate response. Similarly, unless the nurse functions in a role as a spiritual care specialist, the nurse—a spiritual care generalist—should not assume the authority of a specialist and devote the scarce resource of time to completing an in-depth assessment of religiosity. Thus, to avoid potential harm and waste, nurses providing nursing care will do well to delimit the foci for their assessments of religiosity. Spiritual care experts such as certified chaplains should be responsible for any comprehensive religious assessment.

Although the nurse is not to be responsible for a comprehensive religious assessment, it is helpful for nurses to recognize that religiosity does have many components. One typology of the varied facets of religiosity is offered by chaplain Fitchett (1993) and includes: beliefs and meaning (i.e., mission, purpose, religious and nonreligious meaning in life); authority and guidance (i.e., exploring where or with whom one places trusts, seeks guidance); experience (i.e., of the divine or demonic) and emotion (i.e., the tone emerging from one's spiritual experience); fellowship (i.e., involvement in any formal or informal community that shares spiritual beliefs and practices); ritual and practice (i.e., activities that make life meaningful); courage and growth (i.e., the ability to encounter doubt and inner change); and vocation and consequences (i.e., what persons believe they should do, what their calling is). Counselors Faiver and O'Brien (1993) give a very different approach to thinking about the dimensions of religiosity. They recommend assessing cognitive aspects (concepts, values, precepts of religion [e.g., are religious beliefs consonant, functional?]), affective aspects (e.g., what is the duration, source, intensity of feelings related to religious experience?), and behavioral aspects (e.g., any excessive, compulsive religious behaviors?).

Depending on findings from initial assessments, a nurse may determine that a focused assessment about a particular religious concern will be helpful. The nurse may then collect information about this aspect of the patient's religiosity. The process will undoubtedly not only lead to further insight for the nurse as well as the patient. For example, imagine that screening reveals Mr. Lee is a Buddhist who states, "I pray to Buddha when I get sick." As you prepare him for a bone marrow transplant that will require several weeks of hospitalization, you raise the topic of religious coping: "Mr. Lee, I understand from our records that you are like many others—you pray when you get sick. May I ask you more about this so that we can support your prayer practices when you are in isolation?" If he agrees, then a focused assessment of his religious coping strategies will be helpful. Knowing of no standardized questionnaire that is appropriate for Buddhists, you proceed with open questions. You might ask: What other religious practices help you when you get very sick? How might being sick and alone in the isolation room affect the way you pray? Are there ways that we can support you so that you can pray?

SUMMARY

This chapter proposes a process whereby nurses may assess patient religiosity. This assessment of religiosity can proceed after an initial spiritual screening determines the patient is religious. Then, if specific criteria are met (particularly, ascertaining that information about the patient's religiosity is significant to health and health care), the nurse can continue to assess religiosity. Various facets of religiosity exist, and the nurse should tailor the assessment to explore the facets pertinent to the patient given his or her health challenge. Assessing patient religiosity will help nurses to help patients who use their religious beliefs and practices to address health concerns.

PRIMARY PRACTICE POINTS

- Whereas it is beneficial to conduct a spiritual screening that includes assessment of the importance of religion and patient desire for religious support, the more comprehensive and situation-specific religious assessment can occur when the screening suggests further need.

- When deciding whether to further assess, ask: Do I need this extra information because it is relevant to the patient and important for health care?

- Nurses are generally competent to ask patients about only public and semipublic expressions of religiosity.

REFERENCES

Blass, D. M. (2007). A pragmatic approach to teaching psychiatry residents the assessment and treatment of religious patients. *Academic Psychiatry, 31*(1), 25–31.

Cohen, C. B., Wheeler, S. E., Scott, D. A., & the Anglican Working Group in Bioethics. (2001). Walking a fine line: Physician inquiries into patient's religious and spiritual beliefs. *Hastings Center Report, 31*(5), 28–39.

Dehaven, M. J. (2001). Comments on spiritual assessment and medicine. *American Family Physician, 64,* 3.

Ellis, M. R., & Campbell, J. D. (2004). Patients' views about discussing spiritual issues with primary care physicians. *Southern Medical Journal, 97,* 1158–1164.

Faiver, C. M., & O'Brien, E. M. (1993). Assessment of religious beliefs form. *Counseling & Values, 37*(3), 176–178.

Fitchett, G. (1993). *Assessing spiritual needs: A guide for caregivers*. Minneapolis, MN: Fortress Press.

Hay, M. W. (1989). Principles in building spiritual assessment tools. *American Journal of Hospice Care, 6*(5), 25–31.

Hill, P. C., & Hood, R. W., Jr. (1999). *Measures of religiosity*. Birmingham, AL: Religious Education Press.

Hodge, D. (2005). Developing a spiritual assessment toolbox: A discussion of the strengths and limitations of five different assessment methods. *Health & Social Work, 10*, 314–323.

Hodge, D. (2006). A template for spiritual assessment: A review of the JCAHO requirements and guidelines for implementation. *Social Work, 51*, 317–326.

Johnson, W. B., & Nielsen, S. L. (1998). Rational-emotive assessment with religious clients. *Journal of Rational-Emotive & Cognitive-Behavior Therapy, 16*(2), 101–124.

Joint Commission. (2005). Evaluating your spiritual assessment process. *Joint Commission: The Source, 3*(2), 6–7.

Louw, D. J. (1999). Towards a decolonized assessment of the religious other. *South African Journal of Philosophy, 18*, 390–407.

Massey, K., Fitchett, G., & Roberts, P. (2004). Assessment and diagnosis in spiritual care. In K. L. Mauk & N. K. Schmidt (Eds.), *Spiritual care in nursing practice*. Philadelphia, PA: Lippincott Williams & Wilkins.

McSherry, W., & Ross, L. (2002). Dilemmas of spiritual assessment: Considerations for nursing practice. *Journal of Advanced Nursing, 38*, 479–488.

Mohr, S., Gillieron, C., Borras, L., Brandt, P., & Huguelet, P. (2007). The assessment of spirituality and religiousness in schizophrenia. *Journal of Nervous and Mental Disease, 195*, 247–253.

Nelson-Becker, H., Nakashima, M., & Canda, E. R. (2007). Spiritual assessment in aging: A framework for clinicians. *Journal of Gerontological Social Work, 48*(3), 331–347.

O'Connor, T. S., O'Niell, K., Van Staalduinen, G., Meakes, E., Penner, C., & Davis, K. (2005). Canadian chaplains' experience of published spiritual assessment tools. *Journal of Pastoral Care & Counseling, 59*(1–2), 97–107.

Ortiz, L. P. A., & Langer, N. (2002). Assessment of spirituality and religion in later life: Acknowledging clients' needs and personal resources. *Journal of Gerontological Social Work, 37*(2), 5–21.

Pargament, K., Feuille, M., & Burdzy, D. (2011). The Brief RCOPE: Current psychometric status of a short measure of religious coping. *Religions, 2*, 51–76.

Pesut, B., Fowler, M., Reimer-Kirkham, S., Taylor, E. J., & Sawatzky, R. (2009). Particularizing spirituality in points of tension: Enriching the discourse. *Nursing Inquiry, 16*(4), 337–346.

Post, S. G., Puchalski, C. M., & Larson, D. B. (2000). Physicians and patient spirituality: Professional boundaries, competency, and ethics. *Annals of Internal Medicine, 132*, 578–583.

Puchalski, C., Ferrell, B., Virani, R., Otis-Green, S., Baird, P., Bull, J., Chochinov, H., Handzo, G., Nelson-Becker, H., Prince-Paul, M., Pugliese, K., & Sulmasy, D. (2009). Improving the quality of spiritual care as a dimension of palliative care: The report of the Consensus Conference. *Journal of Palliative Medicine, 12*(10), 885–904.

Puchalski, C., & Romer, A. L. (2000). Taking a spiritual history allows clinicians to understand patients more fully. *Journal of Palliative Medicine, 3,* 129–138.

Swift, C., Calcutawalla, S., & Elliot, R. (2007). Nursing attitudes towards recording of religious and spiritual data. *British Journal of Nursing, 16,* 1279–1282.

Taylor, E. J. (2002). *Spiritual care: Nursing theory, research, and practice.* Upper Saddle River, NJ: Prentice Hall.

Taylor, E. J. (2007). Client perspectives about nurse requisites for spiritual caregiving. *Applied Nursing Research, 20*(1), 44–46.

Taylor, E. J. (2010). Spiritual assessment. In B. R. Ferrell & N. Coyle (Eds.), *Textbook of palliative nursing care* (3rd ed., Chapter 33). New York, NY: Oxford University Press.

Timmins, F. & Kelly, J. (2008). Spiritual assessment in intensive and cardiac care nursing. *Nursing in Critical Care, 13*(3), 124–131.

4   Supporting Religious Rituals

Elizabeth Johnston Taylor, PhD, RN

Religious rituals are prevalent. A survey of nearly 55,000 Americans revealed 71% had had a religious initiation ceremony (e.g., baptism, circumcision, naming ceremony), and 69% of those who had married were married in a religious ceremony (Kosmin & Keysar, 2009). Perhaps more indicative of religiosity was the finding that 66% expected to have a religious funeral or burial service. Gallup (2010) polling in 2009 indicated that, 42% of Americans reported having attended religious services at least once during the past week, although 63% stated they belonged to a church or synagogue. Over the past several decades, 9 of 10 Americans have said that they pray. In a 1999 polling, three quarters reported praying daily; those who pray generally believe their prayers are heard and effective (Gallup, 1999).

The idea of "religious ritual" may conjure up images of poorly lit spaces, olfactory memories of burning incense, or sounds of chants or hymns. The notion may also leave you feeling bored or irritated. The religious rituals that come to mind first may be rituals that you experience as meaningless or had thrust on you; or conversely; recollections of religious rituals may be bringing you a sense of peace; comfort; or at-home-ness.

Consider the following questions to allow yourself to be more fully aware of what shapes your memories of religious rituals.

- What religious rituals did you parents introduce into your life? How did your relationship with your parents during childhood affect the way you engaged in these religious rituals?

- As you became a young adult, what childhood religious rituals became meaningless? How did you relate to the religious rituals once they became meaningless?

- What religious rituals do you observe today? What motivates you to continue to practice these? If they are meaningful, what makes them so?

- Have you ever adapted or created a religious ritual for yourself or others? What did you like, or not like, about that ritual?

Reflecting on the impact of religious rituals in your life (or even the absence of such) will help you now to give thought to how you relate to patients who engage in rituals with religious nuances.

WHAT IS A RELIGIOUS RITUAL?

A simple definition of ritual states it is "a set of fixed actions and sometimes words performed regularly, especially as part of a ceremony" (*Cambridge Advanced Learner's Dictionary*). Generically, the activities of rituals are designed to make something special or bring about a good outcome. They may be public or private and participated in with or without recognizing the import of the ritual. They may strictly observe protocols (e.g., Anglican evensong) or informally follow a personally designed ritual (e.g., burial of a family pet). They may incorporate much pomp and ceremony (e.g., graduation) or simple and quiet acts (e.g., private prayer). Rituals typically function to promote a positive outcome but can also reflect psychological dysfunction (as in when neurotic behavior is performed compulsively to relieve anxiety). Because rituals reflect people's deepest thoughts and feelings, they often engage religion.

Religious ritual is a universal phenomenon given that it is well distributed among the cultures of the world (d'Aquili & Laughlin, 1975). Assuming religions are systems of beliefs about the cosmos that offer believers meaningful worldviews, and the concomitant myths, dogmas, and practices supporting and expressing these beliefs, religious rituals are actions that use or reflect religious beliefs. Scientists, however, offer deeper analyses of what religious rituals are and how they function within individuals and societies.

A Social Science Perspective

Anthropologist Victor Turner offered significant advancement in the conceptualization of religious ritual. He defined religious ritual as a process of communication that serves:

> the highly important functions . . . of storing and transmitting information . . . [that is] the crucial values of the believing community, whether it is a religious community, a nation, a tribe, a secret society, or any other type of group whose ultimate unity resides in its orientation towards transcendental and invisible powers. (Turner, 1981, pp. 1–2)

Blasi (1985) accepted that religious rituals involve the symbolic actions indicating relationship between humans and what they consider the divine. Thus, religious rituals serve people by giving them a way to communicate, intra-, inter-, and trans-personally about matters of ultimate concern.

A simple summary of anthropological views of religious ritual suggests these rituals serve three functions (Segal, 1983):

- Religious ritual applies beliefs. These beliefs are about the cosmos (how God and individuals relate) as well as beliefs about society (how individuals should relate to each other). Rituals offer explanations for confusing things in nature and society (e.g., suffering).

- Religious ritual creates or releases feelings. These feelings may be otherwise pent up desires or emotions ready in one's awareness. Religious rituals may allow persons to step out of their rational or intellectual thinking and step into an emotional or expressive mode.

- Religious rituals are essential for keeping people together in a group or society. Rituals express a collective's consciousness and values; by doing so, rituals help a group or society to create or revitalize a group's values and structure.

Experiencing a ritual's symbols for beliefs and the accompanying emotions allows individuals to experience transformation, another major function of religious rituals. Although religious rituals function in these intellectual, emotional, and social ways, people do not perform religious rituals for the sake of these outcomes. Anthropologists argue that they perform them for their own sake (Segal) in an effort to close the gap between themselves and the divine.

In a theory of the evolution of religious ritual, d'Aquili and Laughlin (1975) go beyond the psychosocial functions to biologic evidence to explain the existence of religious rituals. They argue that religious rituals allow people to adapt to an unpredictable universe—a universe with disease, death, and disaster. How? These scholars argued that religious rituals ultimately allow humans to synchronize the cognitive imperative (that innate and universal human need to make answers for existential questions) with affective (i.e., limbic discharges) and motor processes within the central nervous system. That is, to address their existential anxiety, humans attempt to gain some control over the uncontrollable by uniting with an opposite power (e.g., a god). For example, in times of distress, individuals use rituals to entreat a supernatural power for help. d'Aquili and Laughlin posit that myths are created by people to organize their way of understanding the universe. Ritual behaviors (motor activities—always used by humans to master their immediate situation) are used to solve the problem presented in the cognitive (mythic) form. These theorists also describe how the auditory, visual, or even tactile repetitiveness often found in religious ritual affect the human body's autonomic nervous system to produce ecstatic experience. This neurologically mediated ecstasy allows the participant to feel union or oneness with not only the opposite power but also with fellow participants.

Family therapists Imber-Black and Roberts (1993) describe the more obvious or immediate functions rituals play in people's lives. Rituals allow people to: shape, express, and maintain relationships; change by aiding individuals to make and mark transitions in life and make the change feel manageable and safe; heal by helping people to recover from betrayals, traumas, or losses; express their beliefs and make sense of them; and celebrate by helping them to affirm deep joys and honor life with festivity. Although this listing was intended to describe nonreligious rituals, these functions infer how generic rituals have religious nuances within.

Obvious examples of how religious rituals function in these ways can be readily illustrated in the acts of corporate worship performed in a number of religious traditions. Such religious services typically involve music, readings of sacred writings, and messages spoken by the group's religious leader. The attendee becomes aware of inner feelings when the music resonates within or when hearing the spiritual experiences of others (read or spoken). Likewise, hymns sung, Scriptures read and discussed, or sermons preached reiterate and reinforce fundamental beliefs. Sharing these emotions and beliefs inherently means individuals are relating ("fellowshipping"), supporting community. Religious meetings also make evident what the group's values are. Participating in such a service transforms worshippers (e.g., they may gain insight, feel comforted, and more at peace).

TABLE 4.1
Components of Ritual

Component	Examples
Repetition and rhythm (to some degree)	Chanting; drumming; Sufi whirling; repetitive motion as in Orthodox Jewish praying with head bobbing; repeating a ceremony daily, weekly, or annually; reciting a creedal statement or repeating a certain prayer; dancing (e.g., during a Tenrikyo service or accompanying gospel singing)
Special or stylized behavior	Bowing or making the sign of the cross, positioning the body in a certain way for prayer, parading the Torah in the synagogue before reading from it, processing clergy and choir in and out of a cathedral service
Structure, pattern, or order	Following a liturgy or program, organizing who enters or sits where
Evocative presentation	Special garments; glorious music; uniquely decorated worship spaces; burning incense, herbs, or candles; using religious objects that are works of art (e.g., silver chalice for the Eucharist)
Social dimension	Singing or saying a prayer together, eating refreshments after the meeting, "passing the peace" (greeting each other during some Christian church services)

Components of Ritual

Another way to understand religious rituals is to consider what its components are. Various aspects of ritual (d'Aquili & Laughlin, 1975; Imber-Black & Roberts, 1993) are presented in Table 4.1 with examples. This approach to describing ritual allows one to become very aware of the multiple types and layers of symbolism that are instrumental in rituals.

Identifying these aspects of a religious ritual help the nurse to understand why patients perform rituals the way that they do. Knowing the structure and function of rituals also informs the nurse as to how religious rituals for healing purposes can be designed in health care settings.

EXEMPLAR RELIGIOUS RITUALS WITH HEALTH IMPLICATIONS

Nurses benefit from knowing about religious rituals for two reasons. First, the religious patient will be engaging in these rituals. These rituals will bring continued order, community, and transformation to the patient— meaning, comfort, peace, spiritual growth, and so forth. More immediately important to the nurse, these religious rituals may have health implications for which the nurse should be aware. Second, nurses can support patients who no longer can participate in their usual religious rituals to create religious rituals appropriate and meaningful during health challenges.

Prayer

Although prayer is a ritual found in and out of religion, it is arguably the most essential of religious rituals. An academic definition for prayer describes it as "the symbolic utterance of an address toward the ultimate Other" (Happel, 1987, p. 197). Others have described it more colloquially as a conversation with God, or an awakening to God's presence within (Wierzbicka, 1994), or "human consciousness of God" (Leech, 1980, p. 7). A theologian and psychoanalyst proposed that prayer allows "who and what we are [to] speak out of us whether we know it or not. . . . To pray is to listen to and hear this self who is speaking" (Ulanov & Ulanov, 1982, p. 1).

Types of Prayer
Persons can respond to their experience of the divine and pray in many ways. Sociologists Poloma and Gallup (1991) identified four types of prayer experience among Americans:

- Ritual prayers are typically established forms (words, motions) for engaging the divine.

- Petitionary prayers are those that ask the divine for specific favors. Any religious person with a transcendent attachment object (e.g., Buddha, Allah, God) may pray petitions. It has been thought that the difference between invoking magic and true prayer lay in whether the petitioner subjugates his or her desires to embrace God's will.

- Conversational or colloquial prayers are conversations with God. Whether the praying person's conversation is audibly expressed or mentally thought, this type of prayer involves persons talking to God as to a friend (or parent or therapist—depending on their picture of God). This type of praying is common among Christians, with Protestants twice as likely as Catholics to pray conversationally (Gallup, 1999).

- Meditational prayer requires no language. It allows the praying person to "simply" be present and receptive to the divine. The experience may include having words or a visual image on which to meditate on, but it is not necessary. It may involve attention to one's breathing and body position, commitment to putting aside intrusive mental distractions, and a rhythmic action (e.g., chanting, walking a labyrinth).

This typology identifies types or approaches to prayer. Others have distinguished different types of prayer by purpose, including to express lament, confess, intercede, praise or adore, express thanksgiving, and invoke or summon (Dossey, 1993).

Praying for Health
Of course, prayer has been a religious ritual for the sick for millennia. The notion of intercessory praying for the cure or physical improvement of patients (an "intervention"), however, has received considerable attention and research funding during the past couple decades. A Cochrane review of the 10 existent clinical trials (involving 7,646 patients) concluded that "findings are equivocal . . . and the evidence does not support a recommendation either in favour or against the use of intercessory prayer" (Roberts, Ahmed, Hall, & Davison, 2009, p. a). Such unsupportive evidence for intercessory prayer may disillusion some. However, a balanced perspective is given by Cohen et al. (2000): "In prayer, God is petitioned, not controlled; God trusted, not tested."

Although intercessory prayer may not cure patients, how does praying privately affect patient emotional well-being? A critical review of 26 research studies exploring how personal prayer affects health outcomes was conducted by Hollywell and Walker (2008). These nurses observed that prayer (typically measured by its frequency) was usually associated with positive health outcomes (often inversely related to anxiety and depression). This association was particularly true for those who already had a religious faith and regularly experienced prayer. Likewise, they noted research that documents pleading, bargaining, and passive prayers (like wishful thinking) as associated with negative health outcomes. Thus, these authors recommended that nurses not indiscriminately recommend prayer to patients. Rather, Hollywell and Walker recommend that patients first be assessed regarding their religious faith and experience of prayer. Such assessment would do well to determine if prayer is an undeveloped practice used only in times of extremis and if negative types of prayer are used.

Although prayer is generally a helpful and comforting religious ritual, it is important to consider the possible challenges that illness can have on praying. Nurse researchers (Hawley & Irurita, 1998; Taylor & Outlaw, 1999) interviewing patients about how illness affected praying identified the following:

- drugs befuddle the mind, making thought-filled prayer difficult;

- the fatigue, pain, and other symptoms of illness make it hard to concentrate on prayer or attend religious services where communal prayers are experienced;

- hospitalization brings interruptions, and lack of privacy and quiet time for prayer;

- the uncertainties and fears of illness enter the prayer experience, often increasing the intensity and frequency of praying, as well as changing the content and type of prayer; and

- illness can bring to the surface spiritual doubts or distress about the nature of God and prayer.

Indeed, Taylor and Outlaw (1999) identified several spiritual pains related to praying that persons with cancer described. These included doubts about whether prayer was efficacious, whether God was able to respond, whether they were praying in the "right" way, and whether they were worthy or good enough to pray or receive an "answer" to prayer. This evidence suggests that there is room for caution and sensitivity to the difficulties of prayer while supporting patients who want to pray.

Healing Services

The *Dictionary of Alternative Medicine* (Segen, 1998) equates spiritual and faith healing, and defines them as "entrusting the healing process to a 'higher' (God in the Judeo-Christian construct) or other power(s) through prayer" (p. 139). Such a broad definition allows for spiritual healing to include participation in a religious ritual of healing, seeking out a person known for invoking supernatural healing powers, or personal prayer.

Research measuring the frequency of complementary therapy use documents that spiritual/faith healing is reported surprisingly frequently. Studies representing a diversity of adults samples have documented rates of spiritual therapies or healing to be 6%–56% (Amin et al., 2010; Callahan et al., 2009; Molassiotis et al., 2005; Taylor, 2005). The prevalence of spiritual/faith healing use (excluding prayer) in pediatric samples ranges from

3% to 30% across nine studies (Bishop, Prescott, Chan, Saville, von Elm, & Lewith, 2010). These studies indicate that spiritual or faith healing—essentially, religious rituals to petition the divine for healing, are sought out by many patients.

Pilgrimages

A religious pilgrimage is a journey, often made arduous, to a shrine or place of importance in the pilgrim's religious tradition. The goal for many pilgrims is healing, although often a pilgrimage is made simply because it is a religious obligation or search to encounter the holy. Buddhists may travel to several sites across southern Asia, especially to places associated with Gautama Buddha's life. Christians, especially Roman Catholics, may travel to Middle Eastern sites associated with the life of Jesus, or places where saints died or where apparitions and miracles are thought to have occurred. Hindus, Baha'i, Sikhs, Zoroastrians, and others also observe pilgrimages.

A prototypical example of a pilgrimage for unwell or disabled patients seeking healing is that of Roman Catholics traveling to Lourdes, France. It is there that a young peasant girl in the mid-1800s reported having seen the Blessed Virgin Mary (mother of Jesus) who wanted people to come. The spring water from that place where the apparition occurred was found to produce miracles of healing. It is now a sacred spot with several churches that roughly 5 million persons visit each year. Although only 66 cures are recognized by the Catholic leaders as having occurred as a result of visiting Lourdes, witnesses suggest that unwell pilgrims have "mini-miracles" of inward peace or transformation (Stott, 2004). Indeed, as with prayer and healing services, performing a religious ritual is not about manipulating God; rather, it is a process for encountering God.

The Hajj is the Muslim pilgrimage to Mecca, Saudi Arabia, that is required of every able-bodied Muslim at least once in a lifetime. The Hajj is a pilgrimage that occurs over 6 days during the 12th month of the lunar calendar (thus it varies from year to year). Pilgrims perform various ceremonial acts at several spots along a roughly 30-mile route that is walked. In 2009, the Saudi Arabian government estimated that over 1.6 million foreigners traveled to their country to complete the Hajj (Wikipedia, 2010).

Given the incredible numbers of pilgrims and crowding, the extreme heat and challenging living circumstances (e.g., staying in tents overnight, eating potentially unsanitary food), and the advanced age of many pilgrims, the Hajj creates an "amplifying chamber" for disease (Ahmed, Arabi, & Memish, 2006). Hajj pilgrims are at risk for communicable diseases (particularly meningococcal disease and respiratory and skin infections). Thus, the Saudi Ministry of Health offers recommendations for pilgrims that include obtaining certain vaccinations before leaving home and wearing a facemask while completing the Hajj. Nurses can make additional recommendations for Hajj pilgrims such as to bring along a thermometer and a 3-day course of antibiotics and antidiarrhea medications, use sunscreen and seek shade, and maintain hydration and hand hygiene. Pilgrims may also need to be reminded to continue their usual medications and be educated about when to self-medicate. They may also benefit from suggestions about performing rituals during the night and avoiding crowds when possible.

Summary

When enacted because of illness, these religious rituals of prayer, healing services, and pilgrimages reflect a religious person's instinct to adapt to that illness by relating to the divine. These rituals all have cognitive, emotional, and behavioral features. They apply one's beliefs, create or release feelings, and keep connections with others, all the while working an inward transformation.

Likewise, religious rituals performed even while healthy can have health implications. Male infant circumcision, prevalent among Muslims and Jews, does carry risk for hydroureteronephrosis, hyponatremia, penile injury, and heart failure (Hanukoglu, Kanielli, Katzir, Gorenstein, & Fried, 1995; Mor, Eshel, Aladjem, & Mundel, 1987). Religious rituals for healing accepted in non-Western countries but used by immigrants to first-world countries can involve ingesting substances that produce ill health. For example, Sontz and Schwieger (1995) reported they treated a Nigerian patient with renal failure due to "green [copper] water" his church leaders gave him to induce vomiting so he could be purged of his problem. Because religious rituals can have health implications and because rituals can bring adaptation and healing for the religious patient, it is beneficial to consider how the nurse can support religious rituals in health care settings.

RELIGIOUS RITUALS IN HEALTH CARE SETTINGS

A Latter-Day Saint (Mormon) patient for whom you care has summoned the elders to anoint her. A Muslim patient wishes to pray in his traditional way, and he asks you for assistance, or the reformed Jewish family of the patient you will soon remove from life support would like to mark this impending transition from life to death. The evangelical Christian cancer survivor would like celebrate her disease-free status. How can you help these patients to design a meaningful religious ritual? How can you support religious patients who already have established rituals to continue these?

Supporting Patients' Religious Rituals

It is vital to remember that while there are commonalities among adherents of a religious tradition with regard to what and how rituals are observed, there is also diversity. To begin, within a world faith, there are often numerous subgroups or denominations. Furthermore, even within one denomination, there will be differences among adherents in how they practice religious rituals.

General Guidelines
The following general guidelines for supporting a patient's religious ritual will help the nurse to avoid inappropriateness or embarrassment (Taylor, 2002):

- Even if you think you know how a certain religious ritual is performed, ask the patient how they prefer the ritual to be and what support they would like from you. The patient may simply want some hygienic care before the arrival of clergy and visitors for a ritual. The patient may want the nurse to just be present as a witness or may need the nurse's pivotal involvement to complete the ritual.

- Always maintain an attitude of respect for the patient's religiosity. Any internal disapproval or incredulity regarding a patient's religious behaviors, if accompanied by disrespect, can be detected by patients. Respect does not need to mean you share or approve of the patient's religiosity.

- Refrain from offering advice or information about your personal religious rituals unless the patient requests this information and you deem it therapeutic.

- Allow time and privacy for, and provide comfort measures before, religious activities. While some patients may not want medication for distressing symptoms if they interfere with thoughts, others may. A sign on the patient's door can be used to notify staff and visitors when a patient does not want to be interrupted during a religious ritual.

- Respect and ensure safety of the client's religious articles (e.g., prayer beads, religious books, icons, amulets, religious garments). When you see such articles at the bedside, remember, inquiring about them makes a natural segue to assessing religiosity.

- If the ritual requires a religious leader from the patient's faith tradition, collaborate with the chaplain (if available) to facilitate his or her involvement. When clergy or religious leaders do come to visit the patient, prepare them for what they may observe in the patient that could be startling or upsetting for this person. For example, "Rabbi Gold, Liz is on a ventilator, which is breathing for her. She is not able to talk, but can write her thoughts down on the tablet at her bedside. She can also answer 'yes' and 'no' questions with eye blinks." Again, the nurse should respect this impromptu sacred space created when a pastoral visit occurs and organize work so as to avoid direct nursing care during this visit.

Creating Religious Rituals With Clients

Patients are typically in a transition: from healthy to sick, from childless to parent, from life to death, and so forth. Rituals help humans to mark such transitions so that they can move on. Patients experiencing significant losses or changes will attempt to reconstruct meaning and make sense of their tragedy. Religious rituals bring comfort by reminding believers of beliefs that explain or give meaning to life, death, and tragedy. Persons with illness or disability are often isolated in their suffering. Religious rituals, by nature, allow participants to connect with others or an ultimate Other. Thus, religious rituals can be an extraordinary (and inexpensive) comfort for religious patients who are experiencing health-related challenges.

Some health care circumstances beg for a religious ritual. (Think about when the "plug is pulled" or when a limb is amputated or other significant transitions.) Yet it may be that there is no specific ritual from the patient's religious tradition that is appropriate for this context, or it may be that the appropriate traditional ritual is experienced as meaningless by the patient. Either way, there is a need for a new or adapted ritual.

General Guidelines

When planning or adapting a religious ritual for a health care context, it is helpful to incorporate as many of the components of ritual (Table 4.1) as possible. A religious ritual—especially in an acute care setting, does not need to be long, and there may be little time for planning. Having input from the patient or family, however, is vital to ensuring that the ritual will be meaningful. The following points (Taylor, 2002) can be considered when planning a religious ritual with a patient:

- What is it that the patient and/or family want to have or happen as a result? Is it to mark a transition, release pent up feelings, find comfort, or feel close to others?

- Whose needs are important to meet? This should determine who is involved in planning and who is invited to participate.

- Preparing for the religious ritual may involve choosing Scriptural passages to be read, selecting music, shopping, inviting friends, cooking food, preparing special clothing or decorations, writing a poem or liturgy, or other activities. If clients are unable to do all the preparation, they can still determine the preparations needed and who will be responsible for them.

- In what meaningful or sacred space will the ritual occur? If limited to a clinical setting, this space can be made to feel sacred with the presence of a religious object or icon, a bouquet of flowers, with religious music, or (if the setting allows) burning incense or candles.

- What will be the role of attendees? Will they silently support or actively participate? Having a facilitator is helpful. Clients may select a representative from their spiritual community or a family patriarch/matriarch.

- Given the importance of having ways to engage behaviorally during the ritual (as well as cognitively and emotionally), planners can give thought to how this can happen—even for the physically challenged patient. Examples of simple behaviors that can reinforce beliefs include reading or reciting a prayer or inspirational passage or saying "yes" to a statement of faith. Simple behaviors that allow emotional awareness can include following a guided meditation and singing or listening to music. Being together with others, holding hands, and greeting each other all promote social connectedness. An increasingly common method for allowing participants to contribute their thoughts during a ritual is "the talking circle," where participants form a circle and speak in turn while holding a metaphorical object.

- What dress would be symbolic? For example, wearing bright, festive clothing can be worn to express joy and celebration or wearing a t-shirt with a personalized statement can convey a message.

- Ritual participants may want to consider the role of ritual gift-giving. Does the patient want to inform invitees that some type of gift is desired (e.g., a piece of advice, a comforting quote, or a flower)? Does the patient want to present gifts to the participants?

Attention to even a few of these points can help the nurse to assist patients to create a meaningful religious ritual to acknowledge a health transition.

Praying With Patients
In times of extremis, patients (both religious, and not) often appreciate a nurse's prayer (Taylor, 2003). Thus, it is beneficial to explore how a nurse can support religious patients who pray. Before presenting suggestions about how to pray with patients, it is vital for the nurse to observe ethical principles (see Chapter 6) so as not to impose personal beliefs about prayer on a vulnerable patient. Indeed, some argue that it is improper for a physician to initiate and offer to pray with a patient (Cohen et al., 2001; Post, Puchalski, & Larson, 2000); rather, openly praying with a patient should only occur if the patient has explicitly requested this. Given this caution against a nurse abusing his or her position, consider these suggestions for practice:

- Assess in a noncoercive manner if a patient would appreciate a prayer. Although chaplains find "Would a prayer be helpful to you now?" a good question, it may jeopardize the nurse–patient relationship. A more neutral statement such as "Sometimes people want a nurse to pray with them. Let me know if you ever want that." If a patient does request prayer, the nurse can then assess what type of prayer the patient prefers (e.g., "Would you like a spoken or nonspoken prayer?") as well as for what they would like to pray (e.g., "For what would you like me to pray?"). Of course, if the situation is one of extreme urgency, this level of assessment may not be possible. Although a short, generic, well-intentioned prayer may be appreciated, it is also possible that it could cause distress. If the patient has not requested prayer, the nurse can always pray privately.

- Given that the majority of Americans pray using a colloquial style, it is likely this form of prayer, will be that with which the patient is most comfortable. A generic structure for such a prayer that would be appropriate for most monotheistic patients would include:

  - addressing the divine as "God" (even a Muslim would not mind this title)

  - brief acknowledgment of the patient's circumstances or concerns (e.g., "Mr. Lee is facing surgery right now. It is frightening as we don't know what will happen.")

  - entreaty for help, submitting to God's will—assuming this is the patient's motive for prayer (e.g., "God, please be with Mr. Lee in a special way now. May he sense your presence. May what is best happen. May he know that his destiny is in hands of Love.")

  - closing with thanks and affirmation of belief ("Thank you, God. We say yes ["amen" in Christian tradition] to Your will and care.")

Listening carefully during conversations with patients will allow nurses to compose spontaneous, colloquial, and petitionary prayers that express the patient's inner feelings.

EXHIBIT 4.1
Questions for Reflection (Gubi, 2009; Weld & Eriksen, 2007)

- Does praying with a patient change the way the patient perceives me as a professional?
- Is prayer enhancing psychopathology or a harmful faith?
- Am I imposing personal faith and values?
- Is prayer a means for avoidance and defense—for myself or for the patient?
- Is it used to dress a faith that needs debreeding (challenge)?
- Is my method for praying appropriate for this patient?
- Is the offer of prayer in response to a culture to pray with all patients? Is it considered something that should be routine?
- Is prayer part of the patient's agenda or mine?
- Am I using prayer to enhance my authority or power in the patient's life?

- Sometimes when clients begin to give voice to inconsolable suffering, the nurse, frustrated with the inability to comfort, may respond by offering to pray, when what the client really wants is for the nurse to listen, to be there. Nurses should consider prayer as a springboard for further conversation and deeper therapeutic relationship.

To avoid an unethical imposition of religious ritual in nursing practice, it is important for nurses to reflect on their motives and approaches to prayer and other rituals with patients. The questions in Exhibit 4.1 are provided to encourage such reflection.

SUMMARY

Religious rituals perform important functions in individuals and society. They reinforce comforting beliefs, foster inner transformation, allow the expression of feelings, and allow a community to fellowship. For religious patients, rituals (especially prayer) may become even more cherished given their stressors and suffering. Although health care settings may not seem like sacred places for observing religious rituals, nurses can play a pivotal role in creating or re-creating religious rituals for patients and their loved ones. Such rituals will certainly support healing.

PRIMARY PRACTICE POINTS

- Religious rituals perform intellectual, emotional, spiritual, and social functions.

- Prayer is a prevalent and important ritual for many believers. Types of prayer include meditational, colloquial (conversational), ritual, and petitionary prayer. While prayer is often very comforting to the sick, illness can also bring to the surface spiritual doubts or distress about the nature of God and prayer.

- When creating a ritual with patients, it is helpful to consider how participants will engage behaviorally, for what purpose is the ritual, what symbols will be meaningful, and so forth.

- When a patient requests a prayer, if possible, assess for what and how they would like prayer.

- Prayer should not be used to end a patient's expression of inconsolable suffering.

REFERENCES

Ahmed, Q. A., Arabi, Y. M., & Memish, Z. A. (2006). Health risks at the Hajj. *The Lancet*, *367*, 1008–1015.

Amin, M., Glynn, F., Rowley, S., O'Leary, G., O'Dwyer, T., Timon, C., et al. (2010, March 14). Complementary medicine use in patients with head and neck cancer in Ireland. *European Archives of Otorhinolaryngology, 267*(8), 1291–1297.

Bishop, F. L., Prescott, P., Chan, Y. K., Saville, J., von Elm, E., & Lewith, G. T. (2010, March 22). Prevalence of complementary medicine use in pediatric cancer: A systematic review. *Pediatrics, 125*(4), 768–776.

Blasi, A. J. (1985). Ritual as a form of the religious mentality. *Sociological Analysis, 46,* 59–72.

Callahan, L. F., Wiley-Exley, E. K., Mielenz, T. J., Brady, T. J., Xiao, C., Currey, S. S., et al., (2009). Use of complementary and alternative medicine among patients with arthritis. *Preventing Chronic Disease, 6*(2), A44.

Cambridge Advanced Learner's Dictionary. (n.d.). Ritual. Retrieved March 24, 2010, from http://www.dictionary.cambridge.org/define.asp?key=68200&dict=CALD&topic= ceremonies

Cohen, C. B., Wheeler, S. E., Scott, D. A., and the Anglican Working Group in Bioethics. (2000). Prayer as therapy: A challenge to both religious belief and professional ethics. *Hastings Center Report, 30*(3), 40–47.

Cohen, C. B., Wheeler, S. E., Scott, D. A., and the Anglican Working Group in Bioethics. (2001). Walking a fine line: Physician inquiries into patient's religious and spiritual beliefs. *Hastings Center Report, 31*(5), 28–39.

D'Aquili, E. G., & Laughlin, Jr., C. (1975). The biopsychological determinants of religious ritual behavior. *Zygon, 10,* 32–58.

Dossey, L. (1993). *Healing words: The power of prayer and the practice of medicine.* San Francisco, CA: HarperSanFrancisco.

Gallup, Jr., G. (1999, May 6). As Nation observes National Day of Prayer, 9 in 10 pray—3 in 4 daily. *Gallup News Service.* Retrieved March 30, 2010, from http://www.gallup.com/poll/3874/Nation-Observes-National-Day-Prayer-Pray-Daily.aspx

Gallup (2010, March 29). *Religion.* Retrieved March 29, 2010, from http://www.gallup.com/poll/1690/Religion.aspx

Gubi, P. M. (2010). A qualitative exploration into how the use of prayer in counseling and psychotherapy might be ethically problematic. *Counselling & Psychotherapy Research, 9*(2), 115–121.

Hajj. (2010). *Wikipedia: The free encyclopedia.* Retrieved April 1, 2010, from http://en.wikipedia.org/wiki/Hajj

Hanukoglu, A., Danielli, L., Katzir, Z., Gorenstein, A., & Fried, D. (1995). Serious complications of routine ritual circumcision in a neonate: Hydroureteronephrosis, amputation of glans penis, and hyponatraemia. *European Journal of Pediatrics, 154*(4), 314–315.

Happel, S. (1987). Religious rhetoric and the language of theological foundations. In T. P. Fallon & P. B. Riley (Eds.), *Religion & culture.* Albany, NY: State University of New York.

Hawley, G., & Irurita, V. (1998). Seeking comfort through prayer. *International Journal of Nursing Practice, 4,* 9–18.

Hollywell, C., & Walker, J. (2008). Private prayer as a suitable intervention for hospitalized patients: A critical review of the literature. *Journal of Clinical Nursing, 18,* 637–651.

Imber-Black, E., & Roberts, J. (1993). *Rituals for our times: Celebrating, healing, and changing our lives and our relationships.* New York, NY: HarperPerennial.

Kosmin, B. A., & Keysar, A. (2009, March). *American Religious Identification Survey (ARIS) 2008: Summary report.* Retrieved February 28, 2010, from http://www.americanreligionsurvey-aris.org/reports/ARIS_Report_2008.pdf

Leech, K. (1980). *True prayer.* San Francisco, CA: Harper & Row.

Molassiotis, A., Fernadez-Ortega, P., Pud, D., Ozden, G., Scott, J. A., Panteli, V., et al. (2005). Use of complementary and alternative medicine in cancer patients: A European survey. *Annals of Oncology, 16,* 655–663.

Mor, A., Eshel, G., Aladjem, M., & Mundel, G. (1987). Tachycardia and heart failure after ritual circumcision. *Archives of Disease in Childhood, 62*(1), 80–81.

Poloma, M. M., & Gallup, G. H., Jr. (1991). *Varieties of prayer: A survey report.* Philadelphia, PA: Trinity Press.

Post, S. G., Puchalski, C. M., & Larson, D. B. (2000). Physicians and patient spirituality: Professional boundaries, competency, and ethics. *Annals of Internal Medicine, 132,* 578–583.

Roberts, L., Ahmed, I., Hall, S., & Davison, A. (2009). Intercessory prayer for the alleviation of ill health. *Cochrane Database Systematic Review, 15*(2), CD000368.

Segal, R. A. (1983). Victor Turner's theory of ritual. *Zygon, 18,* 327–335.

Segen, J. C. (1998). *Dictionary of alternative medicine.* Stamford, CT: Appleton & Lange.

Sontz, E., & Schwieger, J. (1995). The "green water" syndrome: Copper-induced hemolysis and subsequent acute renal failure as consequence of a religious ritual. *American Journal of Medicine, 98*(3), 311–315.

Taylor, E. J. (2002). *Spiritual care: Nursing theory, research, and practice.* Upper Saddle River, NJ: Prentice Hall.

Taylor, E. J. (2003). Prayer's clinical issues and implications. *Holistic Nursing Practice, 17,* 179–188.

Taylor, E. J. (2005). Spiritual complementary therapies in cancer care. *Seminars in Oncology Nursing, 21*(3), 159–163.

Taylor, E. J., Outlaw, F. H., Bernardo, T., & Roy, A. (1999). Spiritual conflicts of cancer patients who pray. *Psycho-Oncology, 8,* 386–394.

Ulanov, A., & Ulanov, B. (1982). *Primary speech: A psychology of prayer.* Atlanta, GA: John Knox.

Weld, C., & Eriksen, K. (2007). The ethics of prayer in counseling. *Counseling and Values, 51,* 125–138.

Wierzbicka, A. (1994). What is prayer? In search of a definition. In L. B. Brown (Ed.), *The human side of prayer.* Birmingham, AL: Religious Education Press.

5 | Legal Perspectives

Elizabeth Johnston Taylor, PhD, RN

Consider the following nonhypothetical scenarios. Have a guess at whether these nurse behaviors are legal or illegal:

- A nurse offers to pray with a patient.

- A nurse advises a client that his condition is due to "sinfulness" and recommends "repentance."

- A nurse shares with a patient enrolled in a smoking cessation program how the Lord helped her to stop smoking.

- As part of a mandated spiritual assessment, a nurse asks a patient whether or not he is religious.

- A Muslim nurse wears a *hijab* or head scarf to work involving direct patient care.

- An Orthodox Jewish nurse requests to not be scheduled for work on Shabbat.

- A Roman Catholic nurse in a family practice setting refuses to participate in teaching clients about contraception.

As with most sticky issues, the legality of these scenarios depends on the context. This chapter will begin to explore some of these contexts that frame when and if religion can legally be mixed with patient care. Although this chapter does not provide legal advice, it does briefly review significant laws and rulings (albeit, mostly U.S. federal law) that suggest how nurse religiosity and professionalism can legally coexist.

In countries where there is considerable respect for the "rule of law" (where all—including leaders—are subject to the law), these laws often leave room for interpretation. As with religious scriptures and codes, fundamental laws often require interpretation as they are applied because they do not specify exactly what behaviors or spoken words are right and wrong in every circumstance. Thus, in many countries, there is statutory law decided by legislatures (e.g., constitutions) and case or common law decided by judges in courts when it is unclear how to apply statutory or previous case law. To appreciate what expressions of religious belief are legal for nurses as they provide professional care, one must look at both statutory and case law.

We begin by exploring what the law suggests is legal for nurses with regard to patient–nurse communication about religion. Next, we will review how law may guide the religious nurse so as to protect his or her rights as a religious person in the workplace. The chapter will conclude with some suggestions for how religious nurses can avoid conflict with the law while respecting their own integrity as believers and practitioners of faith. To introduce this discussion, we must review the statutory laws that most directly influence whether a religious expression is legal or not "at the bedside."

PERTINENT STATUTORY LAWS

First Amendment

The First Amendment of the U.S. Constitution (1789) states: "Congress shall make no law respecting an establishment of religion, or prohibiting the free exercise thereof; or abridging the freedom of speech . . . ." The "Establishment Clause" of this pivotal law forbade the U. S. congress from establishing a state religion and supports the separation of church and state. It also means that the state cannot show a preference to any one religion. This clause is followed by the "Free Exercise Clause," which prevents the government from limiting or interfering with the expression of any religion. The corollary, it is argued, is that the government should also protect the expression of any religion (Anti-Defamation League [ADL], 2011; U. S. Equal Employment Opportunities Commission [EEOC, 2011]). Interestingly, these clauses can be challenged when considering the very next phrase in the First Amendment, which ensures the freedom of speech, including speech about one's religion. For example, does a nurse's right to speak freely about religion mean that a client's right to not have any religion shown preference is violated? Of course, what this law actually means gets examined in court when two parties disagree about how it is to be interpreted when an individual's rights have been violated. Although the First Amendment protects people from restrictions imposed by the government, it does not apply to private entities. Thus, the First Amendment does not protect nurses' rights in this regard while they are working in nongovernmental workplaces (White House Office of the Press Secretary, 1997); such protections, however, are offered in Title VII.

Title VII

The Civil Rights Act of 1964 not only ensured that nonwhite Americans could vote, it also dictated that employers could not discriminate against employees—including for religious reasons (in Title VII). Title VII states that "treating a person unfavorably because of his or her religious beliefs" is discriminatory, regardless of whether the unfavorable treatment is related to pay, promotion, training, or any other terms or conditions of employment (EEOC, 2011). Religious beliefs are defined as any "sincerely held" religious, ethical, or moral beliefs. This federal law applies, therefore, to accommodation of various aspects of religiosity like holy days, daily rituals, religious speech, dress, and grooming. It also stipulates that an employer cannot force a worker to participate in a religious activity as a condition of employment (e.g., to get a promotion). An employer also must not tolerate religious harassment (other than simple or occasional teasing) or an environment that is hostile toward one's religion. Another item in Title VII allows for an employee who is required to join a union to opt out and pay the dues to a charity, if joining the union is against the religious or moral convictions of the employee. To work to support this policy of nondiscrimination, Title VII also allowed for the creation of the Equal Employment Opportunity Commission (EEOC), the federal institution that receives and legally addresses complaints of discrimination.

Title VII states that "employers must make reasonable accommodations for their employees' sincerely held religious beliefs, unless such accommodation would cause an undue hardship on the employer" (EEOC, 2011). The employer is expected to consider accommodating one's religious beliefs or practices with actions such as offering a flexible schedule, making a reassignment or lateral transfer, or modifying policy or institutional practices (e.g., letting a Sabbatarian nurse swap work days with a Sunday-keeping Christian). Undue hardship includes significant cost, compromised workplace, diminished efficiency, and infringement or burden on the other employees (ADL, 2011). (For example, if a Muslim nurse asked to work in a *burqa* with a veil over her eyes, and the clinic where she worked could demonstrate that this compromised her ability to read printed matter and hence patient safety while administering medications or some other nursing procedure, then the clinic would be justified in terminating the nurse unless she modified her position and removed the veil when it was necessary for safety.) If an employer can prove that an attempt to accommodate was made and that the employee's religion causes undue hardship—and indeed, the employee has not shown flexibility to resolve the issue with the employer, then the employer can legally terminate the employee. What reasonable accommodation means, however, can be debated and is often tested in court. Courts, however, have generally interpreted this to mean that an employer need expend no more than a "de minimus" (minimal) burden or cost (EEOC, 2011; Kaminer, 2010).

Kaminer (2010) also observed that judicial rulings applying Title VII have often failed to protect religious employees because courts have often viewed one's religious beliefs and status as mutable. That is, religion is considered a choice and adaptable. Once religion is viewed in this way, it becomes amenable to accommodation—and an employee can be expected to make compromises with an employer, which it is trying to accommodate.

Religious Freedom Restoration Act

Title VII advanced nondiscriminatory practices "in public accommodation" or nongovernment sectors. Although Title VII applies to employers with 15 or more employees, subsequent state antidiscriminatory statutes apply similar law to even smaller employers. Exempt from Title VII are religious institutions that can prefer to hire those with same religious beliefs (assuming this is required to carry on the religious activities of the institution), Indian tribal employers, and the U.S. government (EEOC, 2011). However, the Religious Freedom Restoration Act (RFRA) nearly unanimously passed by Congress in 1993 extended Title VII obligations to federal government employers and employees. Because part of the RFRA was ruled unconstitutional in 1997, 7 weeks later, the Clinton administration released "Guidelines on Religious Exercise and Religious Expression in the Federal Workplace" (White House Office of the Press Secretary, 1997). As with the RFRA, these Guidelines reiterated Title VII dictates applied to federal government employee religious expression; that is, "when the employees are acting in their personal capacity within the federal workplace and the public does not have regular exposure to the workplace." For example, if a government employee wants to lead a voluntary prayer group at work, post religious material in the workplace, or talk about religion with colleagues, he or she could as long as it was not harassing or creating strife in the workplace and as long as it was not while representing the U.S. government in a public context such as interactions with clients (White House).

Federal Health Care Provider Conscience Protection Statutes

A series of federal statutes provide nurses and other health care professionals with protection against discrimination for having refused to participate in health care services that they find morally or religiously unacceptable (Department of Health and Human Services, 2011). In the 1970s, after *Roe v. Wade* legislation passed making abortion legal, several "Church Amendments" (named after a Senator) were passed by Congress that protected institutions and individuals from discrimination for assisting with or refusing to help with abortions or sterilizations. One of the later Church Amendments extended this protection from discrimination to include any lawful health service or research activity if it was morally or religiously unconscionable to an employee or institution. This legislation also protected federal funding for such institutions; indeed, withdrawing funding was the only mechanism identified in this legislation for punishing offenders (Pope, 2010). Following on the heels of the Church Amendments, most U.S. states likewise passed similar legislation. These state statutes primarily protect individuals and private or religious institutions and not insurance companies or others (Pope). In 1996, the Coates Amendment (or Public Health Service Act section 245) mandated protection for those who conscientiously refuse to participate in abortion training.

A final hour move of President George W. Bush before he left office in 2008 was the publishing of regulations that would extend the "conscience clauses" further. This Department of Health and Human Services (DHHS, 2011) "Final Rule" regulation prohibited funding to those who did discriminate against employees who refused to participate or even offer information to clients about health services to which they conscientiously objected. (Thus, in theory, for example, a midwife who believed that life begins at conception and that life should never be terminated would not have been required to tell a client who asks for "the pill" about alternative health care providers who could help her with her request.) In response to a flurry of legal and sector criticisms about the unconstitutionality of the regulation and overarching, poorly defined terms (e.g., it was unclear whether abortion includes contraception), the DHHS rescinded the regulation in 2011. Although nearly two thirds of the 300,000 comments received by the DHHS regarding this proposal stated opposition to the rescinding of the 2008 Final Rule, most of these comments portrayed misunderstanding of the law and its consequences. Often it was believed that rescinding it meant eradicating conscience protection statutes. The Church Amendments and other similar federal and state statutes, of course, continue to provide the same conscience protection and are specifically endorsed by the 2010 Patient Protection and Affordable Care Act (Pope, 2010).

Universal Declaration of Human Rights

When discussing the legal and ethical limitations of "conscience clauses," the Universal Declaration of Human Rights provides a balance. It states: "Everyone has the right to freedom of thought, conscience and religion; this right includes freedom to change his [sic] religion or belief, and freedom, either alone or in community with others and in public or private, to manifest his [sic] religion or belief in teaching, practice, worship and observance" (Article 18; United Nations). Yet, Article 25 states: "Everyone has the right to a standard of living adequate for the health and well-being of himself [sic] and of his [sic] family, including . . . medical care and necessary social services, and the right to security in the event of . . . sickness, disability, widowhood, old age . . . in circumstances beyond his [sic] control." Thus, this international code suggests that although the nurse has rights that respect his or her religiosity, so also the patient has rights to health that likewise must be respected.

Summary

These U.S. statutes provide substantial guidance for the American religious nurse who wants to legally bring personal beliefs and practices to the workplace and interactions with patients. Although the religious nurse receives considerable protection because of these laws, this protection is not failsafe or complete. The protectiveness of these laws becomes evident when courts interpret and apply them in particular cases as will now be illustrated.

LEGAL ASPECTS OF TALKING WITH PATIENTS ABOUT RELIGION

Can a Nurse Freely Speak About Religion to Patients?

A few cases provide insight into how a court views this question. Two pertinent cases, which were reviewed in tandem by the U. S. Court of Appeals, Second Circuit, in 2001, provide published case law to guide how nurses employed by the government can think about this issue (Knight v. Connecticut Department of Public Health in tandem with Quental vs State of Connecticut Commission on the Deaf and Hearing Impaired, 2001).

One case involved Jo Ann Knight, a nurse consultant for the Connecticut Department of Public Health, whose role was to monitor the provision of services by various Medicare agencies to persons receiving home health care. During a visit to a same-sex couple, Knight and the couple talked about religion:

> Knight said she "experienced a strong sense of compassion for both men and a 'leading of the Holy Spirit'" to talk with the men regarding salvation. After asking the men about their religious beliefs, she told them that "good works [are] not unto salvation," and that salvation was "confessing with the mouth that Jesus is the Son of God and believing in one's heart that God raised Him from the dead." Subsequently, after one man stated he did not believe he would be punished for his homosexual lifestyle, Knight told him, "although God created us and loves us, He doesn't like the homosexual lifestyle." (Knight v. Connecticut, 2001, p. 6)

The men complained and filed a lawsuit, which was later dismissed, but her employer suspended her temporarily and then entered into an agreement with her, which involved removing her from making home visits and asked her to create a "Plan of Correction." Instead, Knight sued. The district court ruled against Knight, and the appeal to the higher court was made. Before explaining the rationale for this ruling, let us review the similar case.

Although not a nurse, Nicolle Quental, worked with the Connecticut Commission on the Deaf and Hearing Impaired as a sign language interpreter for recipients of health care, including persons with mental health disabilities. During one assignment in 1996, Quental talked with the client about smoking: "She told the client that 'the Lord had delivered [her] from smoking' . . . [and] asked the client if she could pray for him so that he might also quit smoking, and then verbally prayed for the client in his presence" (p. 7). A similar episode occurred again in 1997 when Quental was interpreting:

> When the client told Quental she had been sexually abused, Quental informed the client that Quental had "a relationship with the Lord" and "God had helped [Quental] in [her] past dealing with [her] past and [that] he could help her also." She also told the client that she "used to smoke and that the Lord [had] delivered [her] from that." Quental then gave the client religious tracts entitled "Should I Go to Church?" "The Key" and "What Does it Mean to Believe." The tracts contained passages from the Bible and were stamped with the name of a church. (Knight v. Connecticut, 2001, p. 7)

Not long afterwards, a complaint was lodged, and investigation undertaken. Quental was reprimanded in a letter that explained to her that although she was free to maintain her beliefs, she could not share or promote her religious beliefs during time when she was being paid by the state. Quental then filed suit. The lower court ruled in the state's favor, and so she appealed.

Thus, Knight and Quental's cases were considered by the higher court, which supported the lower courts' rulings. In summary, the following interpretations of the law were emphasized:

- In neither case was the state as an employer found to single out an individual for religious discrimination (i.e., neither Knight nor Quental could show that their employer had accused only them while allowing others to share their beliefs with clients).

- The employers showed good effort to accommodate these employees by discussing their concerns and asking for a plan of correction. Apparently, neither employee considered alternative ways of reflecting their Lord's love during client encounters without overt religious language or religiously based admonitions. Perhaps, they both believed that their Lord required them to speak verbally in such a way with clients—an immutable and unadaptable requirement of their religion?

- Neither Knight and Quental informed their employers of a need to evangelize during client encounters (i.e., did not ask for any religious accommodation) when they were employed as they should have if it were indeed vital to their religiosity. (Not that an employer must be on notice for all forms of employee religiosity and be required to accommodate any religious activity, but having such conversations does provide evidence if it is needed later.)

- Although the employers attempted to accommodate, they were also restricted somewhat by undue hardship. That is, the proselytizing created upset patients—an emotional safety concern.

- The primary issue at stake in these cases, however, was the question of whether Knight and Quental—who as private citizens have the right to exercise their religion and speak freely—were, as state employees failing to respect their client's First Amendment rights to not have any religion imposed or shown preference. The government must provide services in a religion-neutral manner.

The court concluded that the adverse effects on the clients outweighed the benefits of free religious speech for the state workers. Therefore, the court supported the rightful termination of both Knight and Quental.

Because this case law was determined in a federal court, proselytizing to patients in government health care settings is illegal throughout the U.S. (i.e., undermines the First Amendment for clients). But is it illegal in privately owned and operated health care organizations? A review of pertinent case law in this regard completed by Panken and Teich (2008) shows that this question has vexed courts. The trend, however, is that when an employee is proselytizing clients, the courts do not protect such activity. It is thought that proselytizing clients creates an undue hardship for an employer: The proselytizing may create safety concerns and misrepresent the values and mission of the employer, effecting business. For example, cases, where an ultrasound technician believed his religion required him to convince a patient not to have an abortion and a telephone triage nurse injected prayers and religious beliefs into calls, were not protected. These health care workers' proselytizing upset clients and showed disregard to for institutional policy, therefore causing their employers undue hardship. Proselytizing to colleagues, however, tends to be supported unless it has caused harassment or substantial disruption in the workplace or violated a policy (e.g., diversity promoting policy).

Can a Nurse Ask Patients About Their Religiosity?

If inquiring about patient religiosity is meeting the nurse's need or simply curiosity, then there is no therapeutic value in doing so. If, however, knowing the patient's religiosity is important for planning health care, then it is requisite to good care. Indeed, The Joint Commission (2005) expects each patient in any accredited health care organization to receive a brief spiritual assessment that allows identification of beliefs and practices. What may be pivotal for the nurse who recognizes a need to ask about religion is that institutional protocol be followed in this regard.

For government health organizations to avoid the appearance of undermining the First Amendment, it is important to have policy and procedures that are consistent across all health care programs (Warnock, 2009). Using religion-neutral terminology during the assessment would also be necessary, as well as making sure nurses avoid any form of coercion while conducting the assessment. For example, an assessment question could ask, "What spiritual or religious beliefs or practices, if any, are important to you now?" This question allows the atheist to refute the existence of any spiritual reality, while it also allows the spectrum of theists to describe their spirituality or religiosity.

LEGAL RIGHTS OF THE RELIGIOUS NURSE IN THE WORKPLACE

Whereas this chapter cannot provide an in-depth discussion of all legal rights for nurses with "sincerely held beliefs" in the workplace, a few issues particularly important to nursing will be reviewed.

Can a Nurse Wear Religious Clothing While Caring for Patients?

Historically, sister nuns have worn habits. Today, a Muslim nurse may wear a burqa, and a Jewish nurse could wear a yarmulke; other religious nurses may wear a cross on a necklace or other amulet around their necks. A bedside nurse in a public English hospital who had worn her crucifix on a necklace to work for 30 years was unfortunately refused the right to continue this practice in 2010. She was told that patients could grab it and that to pin it outside of her uniform was not acceptable. She was transferred to a desk job (Christian Nurse Who Refused . . ., 2010).

In the U.S., however, Title VII specifically mentions religious dress and grooming as an expression of religiosity that is protected (EEOC, 2011). Thus, a U.S. employer must show undue hardship is caused by the employee wearing religious clothing. Although customer preference is never a valid reason for religious discrimination, safety in the workplace is. For example, if the dress or jewelry presented substantial issues for infection control or in any other way compromised patient or staff safety, then this would constitute "hardship." Nurses whose religion requires unique dress or grooming typically can adjust these practices so as to not compromise safety. For instance, a Muslim nurse can wear a short hijab or tuck it into her uniform. She can also keep her arms covered by wearing long-sleeved knit tops under a loose-fitting surgical scrub uniform and wear a freshly laundered hijab everyday to work. Likewise, religious jewelry can often be pinned to a uniform in a way that minimizes its effectiveness as a fomite—and cleaned as often as one's name or nursing school pin.

Can a Nurse Make Religious References to Coworkers?

For example, can a nurse ask if the team can pray at the start of a shift or post religious quotes or notices in the unit? Can a nurse talk about personal religious experience and belief with colleagues? If the praying, posting of religious materials, or personal sharing subjects patients to the nurse's religiosity, it may be deemed illegal in a government context as it imposes one religion over another, undermining the First Amendment (ADL, 2011; EEOC, 2011; White House, 1997). However, it is permissible—like for anyone protected by Title VII—if it is done in settings where coworkers are and if it is done in a way that is nonharassing, does not discriminate against others, and invites colleagues to voluntarily participate. For example, if a nursing team expects and rewards those who join the prayer group that would be discriminatory. Likewise, if scriptural passages that can be interpreted as gay bashing are posted in the break room, that would be harassment. Similarly, a nurse talking about her religion in a manner that disrupts efficiency could create undue hardship for the employer.

In private contexts where Title VII applies, the stance will vary with institutional mission and policy. If an employer finds that the nurses' religiosity is expressed in a way that conveys it represents the institution as similarly religious when it is not, then Title VII would not protect the nurse (ADL, 2011; EEOC, 2011; Kaminer, 2010; Panken & Teich, 2008). Religious health care organizations will characteristically have mission statements (and possibly, policies) that can guide the nurse with regard to what religious messages and behaviors are appropriate in that environment. Again, although nurses have certain rights to express their religiosity at work, Title VII does not protect them when coworkers complain that the "sharing" is harassing, and the employees finds it disrupts the workplace.

Can Nurses Refuse to Provide Care That Is Religiously Objectionable?

As described above, several federal laws and most states have "conscience clauses," which allow a nurse to refuse to participate for religious reasons in an abortion, sterilization, and often other procedures (DHHS, 2011). As medical knowledge and technologies advance, ethical dilemmas increase. Sometimes, religious beliefs offer a response that precludes a nurse from participating in care that uses such knowledge or technology. In addition to abortion, sterilization, contraception, circumcision, and use of certain fetal tissues and fertilization procedures at the beginning of life, nurses may object on religious or moral grounds to end-of-life procedures like terminal sedation, assisted suicide, or euthanasia. Other procedures some nurses could refuse to participate in for moral reasons include vaccinations, xenotransplantation, genetic screening, giving medication for AIDs, and therapies developed with stem cells (Pope, 2010).

State laws vary with regard to what protection a nurse has legally when conscientiously refusing to care. Indeed, these laws vary greatly (Pope, 2010). Although some impose a duty to provide care, others may require it under certain circumstances (e.g., when no one else is available or emergencies), others respect the nurse's right to refuse—either completely or as long as certain requirements are met (e.g., a referral to another provider is made, and care is given until that transfer can be completed). This latter approach is the one recommended by the European Parliament for its member states as they consider the question of abortion care, as it is the approach that respects patients' rights alongside providers' rights.

In summarizing this law with regard to abortion care, Pope observed that those who are more tangentially involved in caring (e.g., clerk or autoclave technician) are less protected than those who would be more directly involved in performing the abortion (e.g., physicians and nurses). Likewise, nonreligious health care institutions have received less protection from the courts than religious institutions.

Although this discussion is limited to the intersection of law and nurse religiosity, much literature discusses the ethics of protecting one's conscience when one is a provider of health care. As inferred above by the Universal Declaration of Human Rights (1948), one's rights end where another's begin. Religious or philosophically sensitive nurses must consider how their rights also carry responsibilities (Dickens, 2009; McHale, 2009; Sonfield, 2005). After discussing the ethicality (or lack thereof) of abandoning patients with health care needs because of provider religious beliefs, Dickens succinctly posited: "if healthcare providers' principal goal is promoting their own spiritual worth through the offer of care to those in need, they may be using sick, dependent people instrumentally, as objects or a means to serve their own spiritual ends" (p. 346). For this reason, ethicists recommend and laws often require that providers disclose their conscientious objections and make timely referrals to competent providers.

SUGGESTIONS FOR NURSING PRACTICE

Given the statutes and stories embedded in the case laws reviewed, the question arises as to how these nurses could have avoided their respective lawsuits while still being true to the dictates of their faith. Could they have? If so, how? It is possible that although something is illegal, it may still be deemed ethical or moral. The converse, of course, is true as well. Although we cannot judge what these nurses' faith dictated, we can draw lessons from their experiences. The following suggestions are offered to nurses and nurse employers to minimize the risk of lawsuits in this regard.

Suggestions for Nurses

- Typically, the cases involving health care workers proselytizing that were reviewed here portrayed clinicians who failed to use principles of therapeutic communication while sharing their religious beliefs and practices. It is likely that if the clinician had not offended the client (i.e., had not been judgmental and not used nonempathic communication), the complaints and lawsuits would never have been filed. Nurses who want to talk about religious matters with patients must examine not only the ethics (Chapter 6) and motivations (Chapter 7) behind their proselytizing but also apply principles of therapeutic communication (Chapter 2).

- Be clear on what is morally acceptable or unacceptable to you in light of your religious beliefs (see Exhibit 5.1 for questions for reflection).

- When hired, be clear about how and why you need your religiosity accommodated. Vague objections are not good enough. If no accommodation is required, then there is no need to state your religion. However, if there is a change in your beliefs that are relevant to your work, make them known to your employer.

- If accommodations are required, be prepared to offer ways in which you can accommodate your beliefs or practices without undue hardship for your employer. Showing an appreciation for what aspects of your

EXHIBIT 5.1
"Sincerely Held Beliefs": Questions for Reflection

- Given my religious beliefs, what health care-related activities would be immoral for me to assist as a nurse? Would my assistance be immoral for me only if I actively engaged in implementing this care or also if I performed work "backstage" (e.g., cleaning the equipment used for an abortion, sent in a prescription for a contraceptive or RU486, or objectively gave information about various other clinicians who could provide the care you cannot)?

  o From what authority or source are these religious beliefs based (e.g., Holy Scripture, tradition, religious scholars' interpretations)? To what extent are these beliefs held as immutable?

  o What are the intended purposes of the religious or moral dictates, which I choose to observe?

- Are there conditions when a greater religious or philosophical principle preempts my religious or moral dictates? (For example, although life is sacred, are there times when it is more important to relieve suffering to allow life to be extinguished?)

- Is it more loving to sacrifice my conscience and support care I believe is wrong than to impose my conscience on a vulnerable patient? How is my personal integrity—hence, my ability to heal—challenged when I go against my conscience and provide care I believe is immoral?

- What are the consequences of going against my religious dictates? (This may give some insight about why we adhere to religious dictates.) Will God punish? Will my conscience be weakened? Will I be socially ostracized by my religious community?

  o What motivates me to observe a religious dictate that may jeopardize my employment or the health of a patient?

  o What is it about this religious dictate that makes it vital?

- Where do my rights end? (Where is the boundary between my rights to refuse and a patient's rights for health care?) What are the responsibilities that I have with my right to be religious?

---

beliefs or practices are mutable or immutable will be helpful for any ensuing discussion. For example, although you may believe it is wrong to take a contraceptive, you may believe it is right to educate patients about contraceptives.

- Know your state's laws regarding religious discrimination and conscientious objection or refusal to care. Your religious denomination likely has legal experts who can inform you about your rights where you work.

- Consider to whom you can make a referral if you cannot morally offer the nursing care in an instance. You may also want to rehearse your short explanatory speech to patients that you would give when making a referral to another provider. This speech, when given in a respectful manner, may be for a client a window into the life of a person whose beliefs and behaviors are congruent and intentional.

- If you are a nurse likely to be asked for care to which you will conscientiously object, have a method for disclosing your conscientious objections at an appropriate time. If indeed your beliefs allow it, make timely referrals to competent providers when you do refuse to provide care.

Suggestions for Employers of Religious Nurses

- Have diversity and conscious objection policies that reflect not only the mission of the institution but also state and federal laws. Nurses are best informed of these policies when they are employed.

- Offer instruction to nurses with patient contact about how to talk about religion in legal and ethical ways.

- Consider a somewhat standardized religion-neutral manner for initial spiritual screening or assessment. This may demonstrate, especially for government health care facilities, that the Establishment Clause is not being breached.

These suggestions highlight the importance of open and respectful communication between a nurse and employer. They also underscore how important it is for a nurse with sincerely held beliefs to understand those convictions. Indeed, much can be at stake—for both the nurse and the patient.

PRIMARY PRACTICE POINTS

- Several U.S. statutes protect the nurse from religious discrimination in the workplace. These include:

  o First Amendment rights that protect the exercise of religion and free speech o Title VII of the Civil Rights Act that mandates an employer cannot discriminate against a religious employee unless it causes undue hardship, and

o "conscience clauses" that protect nurses from participating in abortions, contraception, and other health care activities, which they believe to be morally wrong.

- Proselytizing to patients in government health care settings has been viewed by courts as illegal (i.e., undermines the First Amendment for clients when the government should be providing religion-neutral services).

- Courts have tended to rule against proselytizing employees in the private sector. It is thought that proselytizing clients creates an undue hardship for an employer (e.g., upsets patients creating a concern for their emotional safety). Proselytizing to colleagues, however, tends to be supported unless it has caused harassment or substantial disruption, or violated a diversity policy.

- A nurse should disclose any need for religious accommodation as soon as he or she is hired. A nurse will be expected to negotiate with an employer how these religious needs can be accommodated.

- Many conscience laws require that the nurse make a referral to an equally competent nurse; the nurse must provide continued care until the transfer of care is complete.

- A nurse with religious beliefs and practices that could impact nursing care or the workplace will do well to acquaint herself with state religious discrimination statutes and conscientious objection law, as well as pertinent employer policies.

REFERENCES

Anti-Defamation League. (2011). Religious accommodation in the workplace: Your rights and obligations. *Religious Freedom Resources.* Retrieved July 28, 2011, from http://www.adl.org/religious_freedom/resource_kit/religion_workplace.asp

Christian nurse who refused to remove crucifix loses tribunal. (2010, April 6). *The Telegraph.* Retrieved March 2, 2011, from http://www.telegraph.co.uk/news/newstopics/religion/7560059/Christian-nurse-who-refused

Dickens, B. M. (2009). Legal protection and limits of conscientious objection: When conscientious objection is unethical. *Medicine and Law, 28,* 337–347.

Joint Commission. (2008). *Comprehensive accreditation manual for hospitals: The official handbook.* Oakbrook Terrace, IL: Author.

Kaminer, D. N. (2010). Religious conduct and the immutability requirement: Title VII's failure to protect religious employees in the workplace. *Virginia Journal of Social Policy & the Law, 17*(3), 453–485.

Knight v. Connecticut Department of Public Health and Stephen Harriman in tandem with Quental vs State of Connecticut Commission on the Deaf and Hearing Impaired and Stacey Eusko Mawson. (2001). 275 F.3d 156 Fair Employment Practice Case (BNA) 728, 81 Empl. Prac. Dec. P 40,834.

McHale, J. V. (2009). Conscientious objection and the nurse: A right or a privilege? *British Journal of Nursing, 18*(20), 1262–1263.

Panken, P. M., & Teich, L. J. (2008). *Religion and the workplace: Harmonizing work and worship—some recent trends and developments.* [American Law Institute-American Bar Association Continuing Legal Education Course of Study, SP032 ALI-ABA 1341].

Pope, T. M. (2010). Legal briefing: Conscience clauses and conscientious refusal. *Journal of Clinical Ethics, 21*, 163–176.

Sonfield, A. (2005). Rights vs. responsibilities: Professional standards and provider refusals. *Guttmacher Report on Public Policy, 8*(3). Retrieved July 22, 2011, from http://www.guttmacher.org/pubs/tgr/08/3/gr080307.html

U.S. Department of Health and Human Services. (2011). Regulation for the enforcement of federal health care provider conscience protection laws. Final rule. *Federal Register, 76*(36), 9968–9977. Retrieved July 21, 2011, from http://www.consciencelaws.org/issues-legal/legal060.html

U.S. Equal Employment Opportunity Commission. (2011). *Questions and answers: Religious discrimination in the workplace.* Retrieved July 22, 2011, from http://www.eeoc.gov/policy/docs/qanda_religion.html

United Nations Declaration of Human Rights. [n.d.]. Retrieved July 29, 2011, from http://www.un.org/en/documents/udhr/index.shtml#a9

The United States Constitution. (1789). Retrieved July 24, 2011, from http://constitutions.com/#billofrights

Warnock, C. J. P. (2009). Who pays for providing spiritual care in healthcare settings? The ethical dilemma of taxpayers funding holistic healthcare and the First Amendment requirement for separation of church and state. *Journal of Religion and Health, 48*, 468–481.

White House Office of the Press Secretary. (1997). *Guidelines on religious exercise and religious expression in the Federal workplace.* Retrieved July 22, 2011, from http://clinton2.nara.gov/WH/New/html/19970819-3275.html

6 Ethical Perspectives

Elizabeth Johnston Taylor, PhD, RN

A preoperative nurse admonished a middle-aged patient facing major cardiac surgery that he "might want to get his life in order" and ended their encounter with a prayer. An acute mental health care nurse, while supervising a break, suggested to a depressed patient that "there is Someone who can help. I once was depressed, too, and it was God that helped. Do you know God?" The recipients of both these episodes of nursing care told me these stories. Both stated that although they were initially put off by their nurse's religious assertiveness (or, some might say aggression), they subsequently were grateful for this spiritual care. Both appreciated a renewed commitment to seeking God through religious activity as a result of these nurses' religious encouragement. These stories raise questions: Does the end justify the means? Are there also times when a nurse's religious self-disclosure is not helpful, even harmful?

Caring for patients facing their death may particularly increase some religious nurses' efforts to introduce personal religious beliefs at the bedside. I met a Charge Nurse at a comprehensive cancer center when I was recruiting patients for a research study exploring patient and family caregiver spiritual needs. When I explained the study to this nurse, she immediately asked me to go with her to a quiet utility room. Once the door was shut, she asked me, "You mean it's okay to talk with patients about spirituality?" She was incredulous, happy, and extremely relieved to hear that spiritual assessment and support was mandated by The Joint Commission. Once she knew I was safe, she told me stories of how she had covertly shared her beliefs about salvation with dying patients and prayed with them. Her religious beliefs compelled her to do this, even though she believed she could be fired if observed doing this.

Although I do not know how the patients for whom this nurse cared responded, I am remembering a story told to me by an acquaintance during a cocktail reception that suggests harm can occur. This gentleman told me about his cousin who had recently died in an intensive care unit. "You know," my acquaintance said, "there was this one nurse who was always trying to convert my cousin knowing he was about to die. My cousin dreaded having that nurse!" Indeed, we have likely all heard of clinicians who have believed their role was to make sure that seriously ill and dying patients are "saved." These clinicians potentially bear the burden of not only spiritually saving patients, but also the need to do this covertly so as not to face a supervisor's reprimand or job termination.

These illustrations clearly show nurses disclosing religious beliefs in an attempt to comfort and support healing. Indeed, one of the attractive features of a religion is that it provides explanations, meaningfulness, certainties—all comforting and healing when illness and tragedy raise questions of "why?" and other uncertainties. It is only natural that nurses who want to help patients will share what has helped them. While it may be natural, it is not always ethical or therapeutic.

ETHICAL GUIDELINES FOR RELIGIOUS CARE

Although many ethical models and guidelines are available, ethicist Winslow and nurse Wejte-Winslow's (2007) guidelines for ethical spiritual care are most easily applied to this context of addressing religiosity in nursing care. They recommend the following steps to insuring ethical care:

- To give respectful care, seek to know client spiritual needs, resources, and preferences. Although Cohen and colleagues (2000) argued spiritual assessment should be removed from medicine because physicians are not priests (and inferring nurses are not priestesses), most health care literature legitimizes this process, understanding that health care teams need information about how spirituality or religiosity interacts with health and illness (Taylor, 2010). Chapter 3 describes the elements of assessment and explains how simply asking religious affiliation only provides an initial and limited glimpse into patient religiosity.

- Follow client-expressed wishes. This guideline does not state: Follow client-*un*expressed wishes. It is tempting for nurses to project religious preferences on patients, and offer to them religious rituals or ideas that have helped them during challenges. It is also easy for nurses to essentialize religions, and to assume that because a patient states he or she is an adherent of religion X, that he or she will want ritual Y and believe Z. This directive reminds nurses to follow what the patient requests.

- Do not prescribe your own spiritual beliefs or practices or pressure a patient to relinquish theirs. The primary concern ethicists have in this regard is that patients are in a vulnerable position (Cohen et al., 2000; Pellegrino, 2000). Patients can be easily coerced or exploited by any clinician, as clinicians—by the nature of their role—have the upper hand. This chapter's introductory stories about nurses sharing their religious beliefs with patients illustrate this potential for coercion.

- Strive to know your own spirituality. It is difficult to not prescribe your own religious beliefs or practices unless you are aware of what they are and how they influence your nursing care. Strategies for further understanding the role of religion in your life and work are offered in Chapter 7.

- Provide care that is consonant with your own integrity. Indeed, it is an ethical imperative that nurses respect the religious and other values that they themselves hold (Fowler, 2008). It can be also argued that the degree of self-respect nurses show themselves parallels the degree of respect they show patients.

These recommendations for insuring ethical practice provide a sturdy platform for discussing specific ethical issues related to religiosity and nursing.

PROSELYTIZATION

Proselytizing is the attempt to convert another to one's own religion. Proselytizing, however, should not be confused with openness about one's religious faith if and when a patient asks and the nurse assesses there is an appropriate reason for such self-disclosure. Proselytizing, or evangelizing, seeks the end of conversion. It is generally considered to be morally objectionable to proselytize in health care contexts, even religious health care institutions, if the patient has not consented to it. There is a power differential between nurse and patient, and patients are generally made more vulnerable by illness. These factors combine to constrain a patient's freedom in the face of proselytizing. Ethical perspectives on proselytization as well as nursing codes of ethics provide further guidance.

Ethical Perspectives on Proselytization

Thiessen (2006) proposed that there is a continuum of persuasion. At a gentle end of this continuum is education. While moving toward a more aggressive end of coercion, one passes through advisement and persuasion. This can be schematically presented as:

$$educate \rightarrow advise \rightarrow persuade \rightarrow coerce$$

Thiessen argued that proselytization can be moral when it is nonaggressive and noncoercive; immoral proselytization, in contrast, is aggressive and coercive. Thiessen views proselytizing as ethical or moral when it is done as an expression of care and respect for the other person. It should be done in a way that protects the dignity and worth of the individual. Thus, this philosopher offers a framing for the possibility of an ethical sharing of nurse religiosity with patients.

Nurse ethicist Fowler (Taylor & Fowler, 2011) disagrees. Fowler rebuts this viewpoint, arguing that no matter how soft the attempt at proselytizing, it is intrinsically coercive in a nonreligious setting and seeks the end of conversion. It also subordinates nursing to evangelization, which is not the role of nursing. Fowler would, however, allow that when a patient asks about a nurse's own faith, the nurse is free to share—even as a part of a duty to self to maintain wholeness of person. Such sharing should only occur if that sharing preserves and affirms the patient's freedom and autonomy. In these instances, nurse sharing is at the patient's request, is welcomed by the patient, and aims to support (not convert) the patient. Because such welcome sharing also has the potential to deepen a dialog with patients that moves them toward greater clarity of their own values, or healing, or a relationship that addresses their spiritual needs in the face of illness or trauma, it should not be avoided. Sharing one's faith must be done only with an eye to the *health-related concerns* of the patient, even if health-related spiritual concerns, and not for the purpose of conversion (e.g., "saving").

Theologian Greenway (1993) identified fundamental principles for religious evangelism that provide further guidance for the nurse whose patient has asked for a religious perspective. These principles include:

- *Reciprocity.* This suggests that the nurse sharing religious beliefs and the patient ought to have equal opportunity to share their ideas. Such a stance requires that the nurse is respectful and not defensive. Guidelines for nurse self-disclosure (Chapter 2) include not only initially asking oneself "Whose needs am I meeting by self-disclosing?" but also following up self-disclosures with a question for the patient that allows them the opportunity to respond so the nurse can gauge the therapeutic value of the disclosure.

- *Honesty in both message and methods.* Not only must the message given be truthful, but the means whereby it is delivered is not deceptive. Asking a patient, "Do you mind if I ask you a question?" to gain entrée to share religious beliefs is misleading and coercive. Another subtle way some religious nurses may coerce their beliefs is by sharing beliefs during a prayer, when a patient has only asked for prayer for comfort. "Bait and switch" tactics also become unethical in the context of caring for vulnerable people (e.g., having nursing students obtain patients' permission to survey them about their spirituality, then ending the "survey" with a religious conversation that seeks to steer the patient towards conversion). This principle should also encourage heart-searching among missionary nurses about methods for health evangelism (e.g., is material assistance or health care used as bait for evangelism among disadvantaged people?).

- *Humility.* The nurse who shares her or his faith must not be arrogant or condescending, and not self-serving or self-glorifying. The nurse who is sharing religious beliefs must not be doing it for personal gain (e.g., to gain her own salvation or accolades at church). Rather, sharing must have an authentic desire for the well-being of the other's health.

It is done to please God, not self or others. Nurses who believe they are responsible for converting others are trusting themselves, not God.

- *Respect.* The nurse must recognize that patients are not objects to manipulate. Instead of coercion, the religious nurse should respect and support a patient's freedom to make choices. Of course, this includes the freedom to not discuss religious matters.

These principles for ethical evangelism are attributes important in any nurse–patient relationship. While they are worth noting, it must be remembered that they were written for evangelists, not nurses. Nurses must continue to remember what their role is and the inherent vulnerability of the patient. That is, evangelism that disconnects faith from health concerns and wounds a patient's freedom is not within the purview of the nurse (Taylor & Fowler, 2011). To reflect on how the religious nurse ought to share personal religiosity with a patient, consider Emma's true story in Exhibit 6.1.

EXHIBIT 6.1
For Reflection: Emma's Story

"I held a terrified patient last night for 45 minutes who was hallucinating (auditory and visual) until p.o. meds could kick in. I'd found her wailing in her room. She was in much distress and I instantly knew she needed presence; not just the nurse-in-the-room presence but someone to be WITH her. I asked her if she wanted me to be near her or not. She grabbed me and begged me not to let go.

I prayed silently asking God to comfort this woman and to show me what to do to help. Although it was not an explicitly spiritual conversation with her at the time, it was deeply connected. She squeezed my hands, grabbed my clothes, wailing off and on, screaming at times, moving around, standing, sitting, kneeling. I stayed "with" her. At times held her closely, stroked her hair, rubbed her back, tried to help her slow her breathing. She said "you don't see them do you?" as she batted at unseen demons in the air, adding, "please don't let them hurt me" over and over again. I told her I did not see what she saw but I would not leave her. She asked me to talk to crowd out the voices and I gently, softly talked about things I thought would connect with her based on my knowledge of her life.

As she calmed and regained control, she thanked me profusely. She said it helped more than I could understand. She apologized over and over. I told her this is why I am a nurse, to be with people who are hurting. I sensed I had entered into her agony as she looked deeply into my eyes with that piercing, soul-opening look. We had been present together—heart to heart, spirit to spirit.

In our conversation afterwards, I asked how often this happened and what she did when the voices/visions were so strong, how she sought support. In inquiring about support systems, I asked if faith played a role in her life and she said yes and no. She believed in God and had tried to find a church but never fit in. I told her I had experienced that God loves all people and longs to help us. She said something like, "Yeah, I guess he sent me you." It seemed appropriate, and she lives not too far from my church, so I invited her to my church. I go to a downtown church with a mix of homeless, mentally ill, and folks of diverse ethnic backgrounds. I knew it would be a safe place for her. It seemed the right thing to do. She said she probably would not go but appreciated the invitation (as in this was a gift of acceptance to her, not proselytizing). I suggested she keep asking God for his help and keep praying for her daughter. (She's scared her daughter will develop psychosis as she did). Clinically, we also had a good conversation about why you don't stop taking your meds, as she cyclically goes off and on her antipsychotics." (Emma, RN)

For reflection: Did Emma deliver ethical nursing care? What did she do right? Wrong? Defend your answer with ethical guidelines identified in this chapter. How would you have holistically cared for this psychotic patient? How might Emma's religiosity have influenced her interaction with this patient? How might this episode of caring have influenced Emma?

Nursing Codes of Ethics

While the American (ANA, 2008) and Canadian (CNA, 2008) Nurses Association codes of ethics mandate that patients' "religious beliefs" or "unique values, customs and spiritual beliefs" be respected to preserve their dignity, the respective interpretive statements provide guidance on this issue of proselytization. The ANA *Code of Ethics with Interpretive Statements* states:

> In situations where the patient requests a personal opinion from the nurse, the nurse is generally free to express an informed personal opinion as long as this preserves the voluntariness of the patient and maintains appropriate professional and moral boundaries. It is essential to be aware of the potential for undue influence attached to the nurse's professional role. Assisting patients to clarify their own values in reaching informed decisions may be helpful in avoiding unintended persuasion. (Provision 5.3)

Similarly, the CNA *Code of Ethics* states:

> Nurses maintain appropriate professional boundaries and ensure their relationships are always for the benefit of the persons they serve. They recognize the potential vulnerability of persons and do not exploit their trust and dependency in a way that might compromise the therapeutic relationship. . . . (Provision D.7)

These Codes remind nurses of their primary role of supporting patient health (not religious indoctrination) and of the powerful position the nurse holds intrinsically in any nurse–patient relationship. Sharing of a religious "opinion" can threaten this delicate relationship if the patient did not volunteer for it and if the nurse exploits a patient's request for it.

Although nurses have been sharing their personal religious convictions with patients for centuries, this topic has received meager attention by nurse ethicists and scholars. This discussion offers key points to guide nurses away from unethical proselytization. However, many questions remain for discussion. Questions some clinicians may frequently ask in this regard are addressed in Exhibit 6.2.

EXHIBIT 6.2
Questions and Answers about Nurses Sharing Personal
Religious Beliefs and Practices

Question: But is it not my right to have freedom of speech and religion as I work as a nurse?
Answer: With any right, comes responsibility. While Chapter 5 offers American legal perspectives, the ethical guidelines offered in this chapter provide moral underpinnings. That is: (A) Patients seeking nursing care are vulnerable, creating a nurse–patient power imbalance. Therefore, unsolicited self-disclosure of personal religious beliefs or practices from a nurse to a patient becomes a coercive act. (B) While North Americans enjoy considerable freedoms (including rights to worship and speak as they please), nurses practicing nursing must recognize professional boundaries and nursing practice acts and codes. Nurses are not clergy. They are not even chaplains. While it is in the nurse's purview to support spiritual health, such support does not entail converting a patient (even incrementally) toward the nurse's religion.
Question: What if a patient is skirting around a religious issue. Can I address that?
Answer: Not only can you, but you should if there are health implications associated with that religious issue. If the issue is a deep one requiring expertise, ask if you can make a referral to a spiritual care expert.
Question: Is it okay to ask a spiritual assessment question to engage a patient in a religious discussion?
Answer: While it is appropriate to assess how a patient's religiosity influences health and treatment decisions, to ask questions about religiosity to engage the patient in dialog so as to proselytize is deceiving. The approach offered in Chapter 2, however, provides a potential means for discussing religion. For example, if the patient is discussing his imminent death, the nurse might broach the subject by asking, "I heard you say you wondered what will happen after you die; what are your thoughts about that?" If the patient responds, "I'm clueless and I really would like to know what you believe," then the nurse can share. Again, following the guidelines for self-disclosure found in Chapter 2 will ensure the dialog is ethical. Also, make sure the motives for doing a spiritual assessment are related to delivering health care.
Question: If I am employed at a religious health care institution that openly and explicitly states its orientation, then is it okay for me to initiate religious discussions and offer a religious ritual?
Answer: Yes, if it is within that institution's stated mission and policies. Remember, however, the patient may have not had a choice in what institution to visit for health care and could feel coerced when religion is broached. Most religious traditions would not condone coercive proselytization. Greenway's principles of respect, humility, honesty, and reciprocity still will serve you well.

WHEN PERSONAL AND PROFESSIONAL BELIEFS CONFLICT

Occasionally, a nurse's personal religious beliefs contradict professional beliefs. Perhaps the most common instance of such a clash is when nurses whose religious beliefs maintain it is morally wrong to abort a fetus are asked to assist with an abortion procedure or counsel couples about it as a therapeutic option. As stated above, nurses should provide care that is consonant with their beliefs (Winslow & Wehtje-Winslow, 2007). Pellegrino (2000) agrees and suggests that during initial contact with patients, clinicians should inform patients of their religious perspective if it is likely to influence the subsequent care they deliver.

Both the American and Canadian Nurses Associations' codes of ethics contain a "conscientious objection" clause (ANA, 2008; CNA, 2008). Conscientious objection permits a nurse to refuse to participate in a nursing duty on the grounds of moral or religious objection. Conscientious objection can be invoked for categories of activity (e.g., participation in abortion or sexual reassignment) or for particular interventions for particular patients on the grounds of moral inappropriateness for that patient (e.g., not in the patient's best interests or the patient did not want it). Both codes state that although patient safety is foremost, the nurse must provide safe, compassionate, and competent care for a patient requiring care the nurse believes to be morally unacceptable until alternative arrangements can be made. The patient is never to be abandoned. Nurses can and should, however, communicate this objection in advance. Conscientious objection to participation in particular treatments ought to be discussed with employers (including patients, if the nurse is in solo practice). For example, a midwife may have a brochure introducing herself, as well as a verbal introduction, that indicates how her religious beliefs could affect her nursing care. A nurse employed by an institution that offers treatments morally objectionable to the nurse should opt-out of participation, in writing, at the start of employment. This, of course, would not affect conscientious objection on the grounds that a particular treatment was contrary to the patient's best interests or wishes. Pellegrino (2000) suggests that when clinicians refuse to provide care due to religious reasons, they should assist patients to find a replacement.

WHEN NURSE AND PATIENT BELIEFS CONFLICT

It is possible that a patient may request a nurse's assistance for a religious ritual that the nurse believes is wrong or harmful. How can a nurse respect a patient's religiosity when it conflicts with what she or he believes? For example, a rural Baptist midwife believes in adult baptism by immersion, yet the "lapsed" Catholic mother of a stillborn child requests her midwife to baptize her infant, or a Santeria surgical patient wants a dead rooster to be passed over the sterile field during surgery. If you believe these behaviors or beliefs are wrong, how do you provide nursing care that respects both the patient and you?

Taylor's (2001) steps to creating resolution when nurse–patient spiritual–cultural values conflict are useful. These steps include:

- *Assess.* Determine what the religious ritual or beliefs means to the patient and for what purpose the patient wants to have it. (e.g., Tell me about this ceremony/ritual. . . . For what reasons do you want to have it here now? How would you like it to help you?) Understanding more of the patient's point of view may or may not help to soften your view about the harmfulness of the ritual. Regardless, open dialog can promote mutual respect and help the nurse to begin thinking about solutions.

- *Show respect.* Without showing disrespect, neutrally explain simply and briefly to the patient why you believe the ritual will be harmful.

- *Encourage the patient to respond.* They may have questions and reconsider their position (especially if there is a sense that they do not need to defend it).

- *Continue to dialog.* Identify what the essential symbols for the ritual are, what purpose they serve, and how they can be modified. It is often possible to recreate the ritual in a way that accommodates both perspectives, yet without undermining the meaning of the ritual. Family members (if they share the same religion as the patient) and the patient's clergy can be consulted to clarify what is central to the ritual and how it can be adapted.

- *Make a decision.* Accommodate for religious rituals that are not harmful. Change and provide alternatives for patient rituals that are harmful without trying to change the underlying belief system, if possible.

Note that if the conflict exists only for the patient's nurse, other nurses or appropriate persons can be rallied to assist the patient with the ritual. Often on reflection, a nurse may find that what seemed harmful at first is really just difference and not harm. Appreciating that the Divine can be encountered in a myriad of ways—ways that differ from our own, and wanting patients to be able to have this encounter, can help nurses to support religious rituals that are unfamiliar.

A patient may hold religious beliefs that the nurse perceives are harmful to emotional or physical health. For example, a ventilated patient in a persistent vegetative state has his life continued because the family states, "We want to give God time to perform a miracle" or a patient's ineffective coping with illness appears integrally related to her use of negative religious coping ("God is punishing me" or "I'll just leave it in God's hands"), or a patient with severe pain refuses narcotics because he believes they are prohibited by his religion. Although some of the steps above can be adapted to address such differences between patient and nurse (or health care system) beliefs, this is a much trickier territory to tread. A nurse may inquire, "What makes this belief helpful to you now?" to show respect and dialogue. However, such beliefs are not for the superficially trained nurse to address. Rather, this is the domain of the expert (e.g., a trained chaplain or religiously sensitive therapist). Religious beliefs are elemental aspects of how one thinks about existence. To unskillfully tamper with such essentials can inflict harm. Get a consultation or make a referral.

SUMMARY

This chapter has explored various ethical issues that addressing religiosity in patient care can create for nurses. To provide ethical care, nurses must appreciate the power difference in the nurse–patient relationship. Because the patient is inherently in a vulnerable position, the nurse should only share personal religious beliefs and practices if the patient initiates a request for it. Nurses must remember that their role is not one of clergy or chaplain. While it may be ethical and therapeutic to share a personal religious belief or practice when a patient requests it, it is not the nurse's role to provide religious education, encourage conversion, or challenge the efficacy of one's religious experience. Rather, nurses must be consummately respectful and sensitive when discussing religious matters with a patient (Exhibit 6.2).

PRIMARY PRACTICE POINTS

- It is generally considered to be morally objectionable to proselytize in health care contexts, even religious health care institutions, if the patient has not consented to it. There is a power differential between nurse and patient, and patients are generally made more vulnerable by illness.

- Sharing one's faith must be done only with an eye to the *health-related concerns* of the patient, even if health-related spiritual concerns, and not for the purpose of conversion (e.g., "saving").

- North American codes for ethical nursing state that when a nurse must conscientiously object to providing care, the nurse must provide safe, compassionate, and competent care for the patient until alternative arrangements can be made. The patient is never to be abandoned. Nurses should, however, communicate such an objection in advance.

REFERENCES

American Nurses Association. (2008). *Code of ethics with interpretative statements*. Silver Spring, MD: Author. Retrieved March 20, 2011, from http://nursingworld.org/MainMenuCategories/ThePracticeofProfessionalNursing/EthicsStandards/CodeofEthics.aspx

Canadian Nurses Association. (2008). *Code of ethics for registered nurses*. Ottawa, Ontario: Author. Retrieved March 20, 2011, from http://www.cna-nurses.ca/CNA/documents/pdf/publications/Code_of_Ethics_2008_e.pdf

Cohen, C. B., Wheeler, S. E., Scott, D. A., and the Anglican Working Group in Bioethics. (2000). Walking a fine line: Physician inquiries into patients' religions and spiritual beliefs. *Hastings Center Report, 31*(5), 28–33.

Fowler, M. D. M. (Ed.). (2008). *Guide to the Code of Ethics for Nurses: Interpretation and application.* Silver Spring, MD: American Nurses Association.

Greenway, R. S. (1993). The ethics of evangelism. *Calvin Theological Journal, 28,* 147–154.

Pellegrino, E. D. (2000). Commentary: Value neutrality, moral integrity, and the physician. *Journal of Law, Medicine, & Ethics, 28*(1), 78–81.

Taylor, E. J. (2001). Spirituality, culture, and cancer care. *Seminars in Oncology Nursing, 17*(3), 197–205.

Taylor, E. J. (2010). Spiritual assessment. In B. R. Ferrell & N. Coyle (Eds.), *Textbook of palliative nursing care* (3rd ed., Chapter 33). New York, NY: Oxford University Press.

Taylor, E. J., & Fowler, M. D. (2011). The nurse as a religious person. In M. D. Fowler, S. Reimer-Kirkham, R. Sawatzky, & E. J. Taylor (Eds.), *Religion, religious ethics, and nursing* (pp. 339–357). New York, NY: Springer Publishing Company.

Thiessen, E. J. (2006). The problems and possibilities of defining precise criteria to distinguish between ethical and unethical proselytizing/evangelism. *Cultic Studies Review, 5*(3), 374–387.

Winslow, G. R. & Wehtje-Winslow, B. J. (2007). Ethical boundaries of spiritual care. *Medical Journal of Australia, 186*(10 Suppl.), S63–S65.

7

Integrating Personal Religiosity With Professional Practice

Elizabeth Johnston Taylor, PhD, RN

The worldview of any nurse is likely influenced by religion to some extent. Even the nurse who is nonreligious or antireligious is likely shaped, to some degree, by religious values received from society and family. For example, an atheist nurse may still subscribe to a Protestant ethic of hard work and frugality to prove her worth or use a spiritual practice with religious roots like meditation or yoga.

Regardless of the religious background (or supposed lack thereof) of a nurse, this worldview will inherently appear in the nurse's practice. Thus, the argument developed in this chapter is not that the nurse must divide his or her religiosity from nursing practice; rather, nurses must bracket these beliefs so as to not deliver unethical care. That is, the nurse must try to identify personal beliefs and appreciate their potential impact on patient care and hold these in check as necessary to provide ethical care.

HOW NURSE RELIGION CAN PRESENT AT THE BEDSIDE

I became acutely aware of the potential of a nurse's religiosity to help or harm patient care nearly 20 years ago when I began researching oncology nurses' spiritual care perspectives. For one study, my colleagues and I mailed a lengthy questionnaire to randomly selected clinicians who were members of the Oncology Nursing Society. One of the questions asked the respondents to write about a time when they thought they had delivered good spiritual care. Here is one nurse's response:

> The patient seemed to have unspoken needs. I asked questions to assess the needs. Then I made suggestions, like praying, mentioning my past painful experiences and how God met my needs, discussed different possibilities, and made other suggestions if one was not a helpful one.

This scenario raises several questions: Why did the nurse need to make so many suggestions "if one was not helpful?" Did the patient not respond appreciatively or with some indicator of a positive outcome because the nurse was "on a different wavelength" and shared a brand of religion that did not match the patient's worldview? (What *did* the nurse assess?) Did the patient feel intimidated or overpowered by this nurse's self-disclosure, or did the patient want to be able to talk about his inner experience, but was unable to because the nurse was too busy talking about herself?

Another example of how the religiosity of a nurse overtly manifests in nursing care is from an interview conducted for a phenomenological study describing spiritual care among American Christian nurses. This nurse, employed by a Christian health care organization as a lactation consultant, described her work including spiritual care in this way:

> I'd say 50 percent of what I do is counseling, 50 percent is the mechanics [of breast feeding]. So when the Holy Spirit impresses upon me that I need to pray with that individual, I pray with them. . . .I feel that as a Christian, when the Holy Spirit tells me to pray with that individual even if I'm not supposed to, that the Lord will protect me. I just ask the Lord to lead me to be in tune to their needs, whatever it is. And then I go from there. So that's my strategy, just being open to the Holy Spirit, and hoping lots.

This lactation nurse also described times when she encouraged struggling moms to attend religious services or read the Bible ("stay in the Word") and has given patients Christian literature and copies of the Bible. Her religious recommendations for clients paralleled her own use of prayer and Bible study to keep "open" her relationship with God. Indeed, her nursing was an expression of her religious life, as she prayed daily that God would use her "in a mighty way."

Some readers, at this point, may be smugly thinking they are innocent of such potentially egregious practice. Yet, we all bring who we are to the bedside. The contributions in section II show how religious beliefs about the nature of health and illness can influence how we seek treatment for it. Our beliefs shape how we view suffering and relate to it. Our religious beliefs often influence our health practices from birthing to dying. Unless a nurse is somewhat aware of the vast array of religious beliefs, it is natural for a nurse to assume that how he or she believes is how a patient believes—or should, if they want a belief system that is good.

Although both these examples are from nurses who are Christians (as indeed are possibly the vast majority of North American nurses), the religiosity of non-Christian nurses can just as readily be observed at the bedside. Overt religio-cultural influences may manifest in predilections about caring for only patients of the same gender or a strong respect for preserving the modesty and cleanliness of patients (e.g., Hindus, Sikhs, Muslims). A nurse's religious beliefs may prevent assisting with certain medical procedures. A nurse's religiosity may even impact how she dresses for work.

A nurse's worldview, of course, will also be inherent in responses to patient queries about the causes of illness and suffering or about how to get well. For example, a Muslim nurse's response may reflect a belief that illness is the will of Allah, a part of life that allows testing, purification—an opportunity to seek cleansing and balance mentally, physically, and spiritually. In contrast, a Buddhist nurse might advise a patient to avoid being so enthralled by the perceived self and rather to detach from attachments and to meditate on how to live a selfless life. Religious beliefs could also influence how a nurse teaches health promotion. A Muslim nurse who accepts that breastfeeding is an injunction will emphasize this, for example. Similarly, others may emphasize behaviors their religion prescribes— even while couching these practices with scientific evidence (e.g., sexual abstinence outside of marriage, tobacco, and alcohol cessation).

More subtle, however, is how nurses' religious paradigms can influence their nursing paradigm. For example, Muslim nurse Rassool (2000) describes how Islam emphasizes spiritual care as a fundamental, essential element of care and cure much more than do the Eurocentric nursing discussions of holism. Islam also views spiritual development of the patient as an essential part of healing. Muslim nurses care out of a love for Allah. Rich (2010) shares Buddhist philosophy in a critique of nursing's ineffective use of the concept of caring and a diagnostic taxonomy to distinguish its professional boundaries. Rich suggests that if nursing as a profession instead adopted Buddhist ways of nonself (recognizing that none possess a permanent, separate self, and are self-sufficient), that this stance instead would breed a profession that was selfless. This stance could win the respect of other disciplines for its lovingkindness, compassion, joy, and equanimity (the four virtues identified by the Buddha). These Muslim and Buddhist perspectives on nursing thinking show vastly different viewpoints and suggest how religions can influence the nursing theoretical framework of nurses. Of course, diverse nursing practices reflective of these diverse theoretical framings will naturally result.

While nurses can (and should) respect their own religious beliefs, ethical care requires the nurse to also respect the patient's beliefs and practices. Indeed, to be effective, nurses cannot divide and deny what is an integral part of personhood. A nurse's religiosity can be a tremendous asset when it is not unethically imposed on the vulnerable patient. Religion-inspired beliefs and values, instead of being suppressed, should be examined, so they can exist in a helpful way in the nurse's life and in nurse–patient relationships.

NURSE RELIGION: REVIEW OF LITERATURE

There is a dearth of literature describing the religiosity of nurses and little empirical evidence on the impact of nurse religiosity on patient care. While a more in-depth look at this evidence is presented in the companion book (see Taylor & Fowler, 2011), the most pertinent literature is summarized here. First, a philosophical perspective on the role of religious beliefs in a nurse's practice is reviewed.

A Philosophical Perspective

Dutch nurse philosopher Cusveller (1995) addresses the question of whether religious nurses should allow religious commitments to influence their nursing care. Cusveller raises several pertinent questions: Do nurses' moral and religious commitments stay in the private realm and never enter health care? Can a nurse really divide commitments? Does nursing "professionalism" really require a neutral moral or religious stance? Is neutrality possible? How does nursing care get implemented and evaluated when there are no systems of meaning (philosophy, worldview, or religion) whereby to judge it? After all, science only goes so far in providing answers to what is right, what is well-being, what should be the goal of care, and so forth.

Cusveller (1995) posits that religious beliefs offer religious nurses "control beliefs," beliefs that can guide decisions about what nursing actions to take or not take when universally accepted facts for guiding practice are nonexistent. Cusveller reminds us: "Just as scholars cannot rid themselves of their particular points of view, but have to discuss them in order to develop the best possible theories, so nurses have to bring their particular points of view to nursing and [sic] to discuss them in order to provide the best possible care" (p. 977). Cusveller does not suggest that religious beliefs supersede universally accepted nursing dogma. But rather than sterilizing themselves of religious beliefs while at the bedside, religious nurses can appreciate the control beliefs their religion gifts to them.

Nurse Religiosity

While a few studies can be cited to suggest nurses participating in research on nurse-provided spiritual care are at least moderately religious, there is no evidence about nurses in general (Taylor & Fowler, 2011). One study about spiritual care perspectives among Arizonan nurses' in a state university hospital claimed a representative sample based on comparison with nonparticipants (Grant, O'Neill, & Stephens, 2003). Of the 299 survey respondents, 42% self-reported that they were "religious" while 41% stated they were "spiritual but not religious." Religious nurses, unsurprisingly, were more agreeable about providing spiritual care (37% vs. 28%). Similarly, studies of both oncology ($N = 181$) and hospice ($N = 645$) nurses showed both groups to self-report moderate religiosity and higher spirituality than religiosity (Taylor, Highfield, & Amenta, 1999).

Religious Motives for Nursing

Grant and colleagues' (2003) findings are fascinating also because they begin to explore how religiosity may steer individuals to choose nursing as a vocation. These sociologists observed that many of these nurses, in or out of religion, described nursing as a "calling" and were willing to provide the same services of a hospital chaplain if they received time and training. A study of Iranian Muslim nurses found some nurses viewed the provision of nursing care as an opportunity to worship God (Ravari, Vanaki, Houmann, & Kazemnejad, 2009). Similarly, nurses of other religious traditions may be motivated by an experience of divine Love and wish to reciprocate this through nursing care. Muslim, Jewish, and other religious nurses may simply be responding to a religious calling to do good works. Many religions espouse a "Golden Rule," and this may form a foundation that motivates a nurse. As one nurse put it, "I look to Christ as my example and I look at the patient and [consider] how I would want to be treated in the same manner." For others, the presumption of a divine judgment and potential retribution may motivate their good deeds. As a nurse quoted above stated, "I have to answer to Him at the end of the day." These data begin to portray how some nurses view their work as a ministry, a calling, as worship, as returning an expression of divine love, or as good works required by God. Some from evangelical traditions may see nursing as "an entering wedge" for evangelism.

How Nurse Religiosity Affects Nursing Practice

Most of the research quantitatively linking a nurses' religiosity with practice does so by examining nurse spiritual care attitudes and practice. This research fairly consistently suggests that nurse religiosity is linked with positive attitudes toward providing spiritual care, which is directly related to the frequency of giving spiritual care (e.g., Chan, 2009; Grant, O'Neil, & Stephens, 2003; Musgrave & McFarlane, 2004; Taylor, 2005).

Other research identifying what nurses view as appropriate spiritual care practice indicates nurses typically include religious practices and discussions as spiritual care "interventions" (e.g., Cavendish et al., 2003; Sellers & Haag, 1998). Although this body of evidence is often collected from American parish nurses as well as nurses who are keen to participate in such research, it is still instructive to learn that nurses pray with and for patients, read holy scriptures, offer other religious resources (e.g., books, videos, religious music), support patient religious rituals as needed, and have conversations with patients about religious or spiritual matters. Pesut and Reimer-Kirkham's (2009) ethnographic study describes how Canadian nurses sometime use their religious experience as a connecting point with patients—a way to gain entrée to talk with them about spirituality, whereas at other times, it is something to hold back.

A detailed review of the evidence completed by Gielen and colleagues (2009) supported the hypothesis that nurse religiosity and world view does influence attitudes toward euthanasia and physician-assisted suicide. Religious affiliation and doctrine, observance of religious practices, and the personal importance of religion were found to be factors influencing attitude.

Qualitative studies from Canada, Sweden, and the United States briefly portray how nurses' religions help them to maintain hope, find comfort, cope with the stressors of work, and provide a meaningful orientation (Burkhart & Hogan, 2008; Duggleby, Cooper, & Penz, 2009; Ekedahl & Wengström, 2009; Geller, Micco, Silver, et al., 2009). Because religions offer individuals ways of understanding suffering, explaining life and death, purpose for living, and guidance in clinical moral decisions, religious nurses have a framework for making sense of the tragedies they continually witness at work. Religions characteristically also provide believers with hope, social support, and practices that promote emotional and physical health (Levine, 2001). If a nurse does find these benefits from a religion, she or he undoubtedly has an important asset for dealing with the stressors of nursing practice.

This scanty evidence about nurses' religiosity may mirror that observed among patients: that is, a solid intrinsic religiosity (i.e., lived and integrated religion) is associated with positive outcomes, whereas extrinsic religiosity (i.e., goal-oriented religion) may not be helpful (Christopher, 2010; Musgrave & McFarlane, 2004). Similarly, one person's religious experience may simultaneously contain helpful and unhelpful beliefs, producing positive and negative religious coping. Research findings indicate that positive religious beliefs are associated with positive outcomes, and negative religious beliefs are linked to negative outcomes (e.g., Ano & Vasconcelles, 2005; Bunta, 2009). Thus, it is likely that it is the nurse with high intrinsic religiosity and a paucity of negative religious beliefs who is well equipped for the rigors of nursing.

NURSE RELIGION AT THE BEDSIDE: PERSONAL AND PROFESSIONAL IMPLICATIONS

For the nurse with a religious orientation, it is imperative that he or she be aware of this religiosity so that how it influences nursing care can be understood. Only then can it be bracketed so that ethical nursing care can be given. Perhaps the two mandates offered in this section might better be labeled "Know Thyself" and "Know Thy Power on Patients."

Improving Self-Awareness

Recognizing how your own religious beliefs might influence your nursing care requires that you have an awareness of what your beliefs are. Just as one Buddhist patient will interpret and apply Buddhist beliefs differently than another Buddhist patient, so you as a nurse may have different perspectives from others in your religious tradition. For example, you may accept only 70% of your denomination's doctrines or accept all of them but in your own unique way, or you may have been raised X, converted to Y, but now worship with adherents of Z or an interdenominational congregation. Regardless, appreciating what your unique religious beliefs and practices are and how they have an impact on you as a nurse is essential.

Questions for your personal reflection are offered in Exhibit 7.1 to allow you to progress on your journey toward greater awareness in this regard. You may find doing such independent inner work is facilitated by writing in a journal or by walking while you think. Another way to gain insight into your own religiosity is to complete a questionnaire or research instrument that measures some aspect of religiosity (e.g., the Brief RCOPE; (Pargament, Feuille, & Burdzy, 2011), which measures positive and negative religious coping and is available for free online at http://www.mdpi.com/2077-1444/2/i/51/pdf).

These suggestions for "knowing thyself" can be done alone. However, you may find it beneficial to interact with someone trained to help you explore your religious experience, especially if you find that the journey of self-discovery is challenging or frightening. Trained or trustworthy clergy can help you understand a religious tradition's doctrines and ways of living. Trained spiritual directors can also be enormously helpful for exploring personal religiosity. Spiritual directors (or soul friends or holy listeners) can be located at retreat centers or online at the Spiritual Directors International website (www.sdiworld.org). More information is available at this website about who spiritual directors are and what they do.

EXHIBIT 7.1
My Religiosity: Questions for Reflection

- What religion/s or philosophical perspective shape me most? What religious beliefs do I keep from my family of origin? From my extended family? From my present partner/family? From school and society?
- How have these beliefs changed over my lifetime? Why? Any changes in my religiosity due to adversity?
- How strongly do I hold to my religious beliefs? (1 = hanging on them by a thread, 10 = they represent complete truth to me) How receptive (or afraid) am I toward evaluating my beliefs?
- What do I believe about an Ultimate Other (whatever is divine or sacred)? How is this entity (or entities) personally involved in human lives? In my life?
- What religious beliefs do I have about the causes and treatments for disease and suffering?
- What do I believe about death and afterlife?
- How meaningful are my religious practices? (1 = I just go through the motions, 10 = my spirit is often nourished by them)
- How does being a nurse, witnessing suffering and transformation in patients, affect my religiosity?

Understanding the Impact of Nurse Religiosity on Patients

A nurse's religiosity can have an extremely powerful effect on a patient, for better or for worse. Thus, once a nurse appreciates what his or her religiosity is, it is essential to consider how this religiosity might be present in the nurse–patient relationship. To begin this exploration, consider the questions in Exhibit 7.2. Writing your ruminations in a journal may be helpful.

Another method in increasing your awareness of how your religiosity presents itself in patient care is to do a process recording where you write down verbatim what you and a patient said during a dialog (as best as you can, soon after the encounter, if possible). This is a common strategy used by chaplains. Just reading over such a recording may immediately allow you to recognize the nontherapeutic aspects of your words. You can pose questions of the dialog like: Where did I try to steer or control the conversation? Where did I run away from emotional/spiritual/religious pain or change the topic? What motivated me to say . . .? (See Chapter 2.)

Another source of information about how religiosity has positively or negatively influenced the therapeutic effectiveness of the nurse–patient

---

EXHIBIT 7.2
How My Religiosity Impacts My Nursing: Questions for Reflection

---

- How might my beliefs about the Divine impact my interactions with nontheistic patients? If nontheistic: How do my beliefs about the absence or impotence of any divinity affect the way I relate to patients who believe in a god?
- How do my religious beliefs about the causes and treatments for disease and suffering influence how I take care of my own health? How does how I take care of my own health influence how I care for the health of others? How do my beliefs influence what I say to comfort patients who are suffering?
- How do my beliefs about death and afterlife potentially influence the words I use to comfort the dying and bereaved?
- Considering how meaningful or meaningless my religious practices are, how does my experience influence my reactions to patients' use of religious practices (e.g., prayer)?
- When a patient holds to religious beliefs or practices that I believe are unhelpful or harmful, what is my inner and expressed response? How might this response affect my nursing care? (e.g., Make me more controlling of the conversation? More apt to physically or emotionally run away [change the subject]?)
- Did religious motives influence my decision to become a nurse? If so, how do these religious motives fare when the work gets morally distressing, or when I feel compassion fatigue or feel ineffective?
- How does my religion or philosophical perspective nourish me as a nurse? What specific times can I remember of when my religious beliefs or practices particularly helped me in my nursing?

---

relationship can come from patients themselves! An introduction of a religious topic in conversation, for example, may produce a telling nonverbal response (e.g., face may become more rigid, eyes avert, or body turns away). More likely, the polite patient may simply change the topic or offer a superficial answer indicating disinterest in pursuing the topic further.

Potential Pitfalls

Some religious traditions include a strong mandate to evangelize others, or a nurse's experience of the Divine may be so intensely positive, this nurse is eager to tell others so that they, too, can have this experience. However, unethical religious proselytizing never comes from patient need and always from a nurse's need (Chapter 6). Given the vulnerable position of patients and that salvation is not usually a matter of health—the domain of nurses—it is highly unlikely that nursing care will require an overt presentation of a religion's gospel. While it may sometimes be appropriate to self-disclose personal religious beliefs, it should be done only while following patient cues.

In addressing the question of whether spiritual care allows for Christian evangelism, Taylor (2011) observes the import of nurse reflection. The following questions can guide:

- Is it my responsibility to ensure salvation as I know it for all patients (or at least dying ones for whom I care)? Do I have a "savior complex?" Do I really trust God to do the saving? Christian nurses will readily realize that it is God who does the saving. Furthermore, a loving God is a God of free choice that does not coerce vulnerable humans to faith. Religious nurses will do well if they consider in what ways they may steer conversations with patients for the purpose of religious proselytization.

- Am I able to accept all as children of God? Am I able to value varied forms of religious experience and expression, or do I think that my religion has the market on truth and salvation? Such a view may portray a small, narrow view of God.

- What is the source of what I share? My gut or intuition? Holy Spirit? Has God (vs. inner need) prompted me to share with this particular patient? Many religious nurses sense a divine prompting to initiate religious discourse or offer prayer. While a nurse should never defer such promptings, it is likely often the case that such "promptings" are actually reflective of the nurse's personal need. A God who recognizes freedom as a requisite of love does not model a coercive proselytization. Awareness of the interplay between God and self is pivotal to making sense of such promptings.

- Do I want to share my beliefs because of a personal need or to meet a patient's need? Sometimes, a nurse wanting to share personal beliefs does so because of a tacit assumption (or fear) that "everyone should be like me!" It may even be possible that desire for recognition in one's religious community or anticipation of a reward in the afterlife may prompt proselytization. Honest reflection on the part of the nurse is necessary if such self-centeredness prompts evangelism.

- Have I spoken the gospel by my actions so that I have earned the right to speak in words? This question refers to the need for an established respectful nurse–patient relationship that leads a patient to inquire of a nurse about her religiosity. Only when a nurse has earned this respect, and a patient trusts enough to broach a religious topic, is the nurse ethically permitted to self-disclose after receiving a cue. Guidelines for self-disclosure presented in Chapter 2 should then be followed.

These questions can guide a nurse from falling into the potential pit of preaching "good news" that becomes bad news.

Psychotherapist Case (1997) identified additional phenomena that can create pitfalls for religious clinicians. In addition to being a "missionary" (when work is a context for proselytizing) and seeing "My way is Yahweh" (when the clinician poses as expert in spiritual matters, failing to recognize a diversity of valid perspectives), these pitfalls—actually types of countertransference—include:

- sibling complex (when there is excessive agreement or loose interpretations because of the clinician's religious experience has much in common with the patient's)

- being a spiritualizer (when the clinician views all issues as needing a spiritual antidote, even when other interventions may be more appropriate)

- being reactionary (when there is an angry or defiant reaction toward the religious patient), and

- window shopping (when curiosity motivates the clinician to inquire about a patient's religiosity or wants to gratify personal need—possibly due to personal restrictive religiosity).

These observations alert any religious nurse to the myriad of ways that personal religiosity can manifest in the nurse–patient encounter.

CONCLUSION

Many nurses are religious. The religious dimension of personhood cannot be extracted and placed in the nurse's locker while she or he works. Indeed, a small body of evidence indicates nurse religiosity is related to attitudes and practice, especially about spiritual care and end-of-life care. It is important for nurses to reflect on how their personal religiosity does have an impact on their provision of care. Without this bracketing, it is inevitable that the nurse's religiosity will manifest in disrespectful and harmful ways at the bedside.

PRIMARY PRACTICE POINTS

- Regardless of the religious background (or supposed lack thereof) of a nurse, this worldview will inherently appear in the nurse's practice. Therefore, the nurse must try to recognize personal beliefs and appreciate their potential impact on patient care and hold these in check as necessary to provide ethical care.

- Nursing research begins to offer evidence that a nurse's religiosity often motivates care. It also starts to show how a nurse's religiosity affects ethical decision making, nurse–patient conversation, and what nursing care is provided.

- Unexamined religious influences on nursing care can lead to potential pitfalls such as a "savior (or missionary) complex," spiritualizing every patient problem, nontherapeutic curiosity, and failure to appreciate the validity of diverse worldviews.

REFERENCES

Ano, G. G., & Vasconcelles, E. B. (2005). Religious coping and psychological adjustment to stress: A meta-analysis. *Journal of Clinical Psychology, 61,* 461–480.

Bunta, A. (2009). A study of anxiety, religious coping, and selected predictor variables in emergency room and intensive care unit nurses at a hospital in Phoenix, Arizona. *Dissertation Abstracts International: Section B: The Sciences and Engineering, 69*(12-B), 7841.

Burkhart, L., & Hogan, N. (2008). An experiential theory of spiritual care in nursing practice. *Qualitative Health Research, 18,* 928–938.

Case, P. W. (1997). Potential sources of countertransference among religious therapists. *Counseling and Values, 41,* 97–107.

Cavendish, R., Konecny, L., Luise, B. K., & Lanza, M. (2004). Nurses enhance performance through prayer. *Holistic Nursing Practice, 18,* 26–31.

Cavendish, R., Konecny, L., Mitzeliotis, C., Russo, D., Luise, B., Lanza, M., Medefindt, J., & Bajo, M. A. (2003). Spiritual care activities of nurses using Nursing Interventions Classification (NIC) labels. *International Journal of Nursing Terminology Classification, 14*(4), 113–124.

Chan, M. F. (2009). Factors affecting nursing staff in practicing spiritual care. *Journal of Clinical Nursing, 19*(15–16), 2128–2136.

Christopher, S. A. (2010). The relationship between nurses' religiosity and willingness to let patients control the conversation about end-of-life care. *Patient Education and Counseling, 78,* 250–255.

Cusveller, B. S. (1995). A view from somewhere: The presence and function of religious commitment in nursing practice. *Journal of Advanced Nursing, 22,* 973–978.

Duggleby, W., Cooper, D., & Penz, K. (2009). Hope, self-efficacy, spiritual well-being and job satisfaction. *Journal of Advanced Nursing, 65,* 2376–2385.

Ekedahl, M. A., & Wengström, Y. (2010). Caritas, spirituality and religiosity in nurses' coping. *European Journal of Cancer Care, 19*(4), 530–537.

Geller, G., Micco, E., Silver R. J., Kolodner, K., & Bernhardt, B. A. (2009). The role and impact of personal faith and religion among genetic service providers. *American Journal of Medical Genetics. Part C: Seminars in Medical Genetics, 151C*(1), 31–40.

Gielen, J., van den Branden, S., van Iersel, T., & Broeckaert, B. (2009). Religion, world view and the nurse: Results of a quantitative survey among Flemish palliative care nurses. *International Journal of Palliative Nursing, 15,* 590–599.

Grant, D., O'Neil, K. M., & Stephens, L. S. (2003). Neosecularization and craft versus professional religious authority in a nonreligious organization. *Journal for the Scientific Study of Religion, 43,* 479–487.

Musgrave, C. F., & McFarlane, E. A. (2004b). Israeli oncology nurses' religiosity, spiritual well-being, and attitudes toward spiritual care: A path analysis. *Oncology Nursing Forum, 31,* 321–327.

Pargament, K., Feuille, M., & Burdzy, D. (2011). The brief RCOPE: Current psychometric status of a short measure of religious coping. *Religions, 2,* 51–76.

Pesut, B., & Reimer-Kirkham, S. (2009). Situated clinical encounters in the negotiation of religious and spiritual plurality: A critical ethnography. *International Journal of Nursing Studies, 47*(7), 815–825.

Rassool, G. H. (2000). The crescent and Islam: Healing, nursing and the spiritual dimension. Some considerations towards an understanding of the Islamic perspectives on caring. *Journal of Advanced Nursing, 32,* 1476–1484.

Ravari, A., Vanaki, Z., Houmann, H., & Kazemnejad, A. (2009). Spiritual job satisfaction in an Iranian nursing context. *Nursing Ethics, 16*(1), 19–30.

Rich, K. L. (2010). No essence no self: Using a Buddhist perspective to characterize the nature of nursing. *Advances in Nursing Science, 33,* 344–351.

Sellers, S. C., & Haag, B. A. (1998). Spiritual nursing interventions. *Journal of Holistic Nursing, 16,* 338–354.

Taylor, E. J. (2005). Spiritual care nursing research: The state of the science. *Journal of Christian Nursing, 22*(1), 22–28.

Taylor, E. J. (2011). Spiritual care: Evangelism at the bedside? *Journal of Christian Nursing, 28*(4), 194–202.

Taylor, E. J., & Fowler, M. D. (2011). The nurse as a religious person. In M. D. Fowler, S. Reimer-Kirkham, R. Sawatzky, & E. J. Taylor (Eds.), *Religion, religious ethics, and nursing* (pp. 339–357). New York, NY: Springer Publishing Company.

Taylor, E. J., Highfield, M. F., & Amenta, M. O. (1999). Predictors of oncology and hospice nurses' spiritual care perspectives and practices. *Applied Nursing Research, 12*(1), 30–37.

Religions: Beliefs, Practices, and Nursing Implications

INTRODUCTION

Although several nursing textbooks offer condensed information about diverse religions, they fail to provide any social and theological context for that information. Sometimes, the facts listed are incorrect—or at least, for some adherents. Indeed, a factoid approach to describing religions essentializes religions, reducing them to oversimplified facts that are not always applicable to all adherents. This section attempts to correct for these limitations, while still making an abundance of information accessible for the nurse. This information about numerous religions is found in the following chapters.

Although these chapters provide nurses with a rich perspective on the beliefs and practices patients from diverse religions may observe, the nurse must remember that he or she is not the expert or authority. While preparing the Christian Orthodox chapter, emails with Contributor Reverend John Matusiak brought this point to the fore. Matusiak illustrates this: "An Orthodox patient is in hospital. On Thursday night he fills in his meal preferences for Friday, understanding that he is not fully bound to the fasting practices, so he orders ham. What is the nurse to do? Tell him he can't have the ham because, as an Orthodox Christian, he's not supposed to eat meat on a Friday? Imagine the priest coming in on Friday, seeing an uneaten ham dinner, asking why the patient didn't eat, and having the patient respond, 'because the staff reminded me that Orthodox Christians don't eat meat on Fridays.'" Indeed, this would be odd. Although it is hard to think any nurse would consider it ethical to tell a patient how to observe his or her religion, it is a point well taken. These pages synthesize generations (even millennia) of a religion's beliefs and practices. It is the clergy who are equipped to interpret theology and guide patient religiosity. The nurse's role is that of witness, advocate, facilitator, and supporter of patient religiosity.

Each chapter presents a broad brush stroke about a religion (or cluster of related religions). Although the chapters present resources for further information, you may also find leads to further information about more obscure religious traditions as well as prominent ones from the following websites:

- The Association of Religion Data Archives' (ARDA) "American Denominations: Profiles" (http://www.thearda.com/Denoms/families/index.asp)

- The Hartford Institute for Religion Research's "Official Denominational Web Sites" (http://hirr.hartsem.edu/denom/homepages.html), or

- The University of Virginia's "Alphabetic Listing of Group Profile Pages" (http://classic-web.archive.org/web/20060902232910/religiousmove ments.lib.virginia.edu/profiles/listalpha.htm) or "Links to Religious Bodies Organized According to J. Gordon Melton's Religious Family Groupings" (http://classic-web.archive.org/web/20060829045724/religiousmovements.lib.virginia.edu/profiles/listmelton.htm).

Of course, the best source of information about how a particular patient or family carer believes and practices a religion is that patient or family member. It is vital that a nurse never assumes that a patient accepts all the tenets of a religion or interprets these tenets as do others. Therefore, the following tables profiling prevalent first-world religions are offered here to provide an introductory foundation for the nurse who is caring for a religious patient. It is essential, however, that nurses always assume a humble curiosity about another's religiosity.

8

Anabaptist-Descended Groups: Amish, Brethren, Hutterites, and Mennonites

CONTRIBUTOR: *Joseph J. Kotva, Jr., PhD*
NURSE REVIEWER: *Anna Frances Z. Wenger, PhD, RN, FAAN*

Theology and Social History

Mennonites, Brethren, Amish, and Hutterite communities are the main heirs of the radical end of 16th century Protestant Reformation. Beginning in Zürich, Switzerland, the movement claimed that the reformers were not radical enough in their use of Scripture to criticize church practices. A key element in this radical reformation critique was the insistence that baptism be reserved for confessing adults, given infants and children were not ready to repent and promise to live lives of costly discipleship. Derided as "Anabaptists," re-baptizers, the movement was declared illegal and its adherents severely persecuted.

The eventual spread of Mennonites across Europe and then North America, South America, and Africa was originally driven by both a deep evangelistic sense and the reality of fleeing periodic persecution. Persecution, along with the conviction that the church is to be demonstrably and visibly distinct from the world, led to a lengthy period of being "the quiet in the land"—somewhat isolated communities that were often admired by outsiders for their disciplined lives of mutual support and accountability. In the second half of the 20th century, there was a rebirth of evangelistic zeal among many Mennonite groups, which is particularly visible throughout Africa.

In North America, most Mennonite groups no longer live in visibly distinct communities, although Amish, Hutterites, and various "conservative" Mennonite groups still live in tight-knit groups. Anabaptists place a premium on the life and teachings of Jesus, especially the Sermon on the Mount, for the life and practice of both individual Christians and for the gathered life of the church. Most North American Mennonites value higher education and gravitate toward professions that are seen as being of service to the wider human community (e.g., teachers, health care workers, social workers). By contrast, the Amish usually end formal education with the 8th grade. While most Mennonite groups participate in health insurance, the Amish eschew secular insurance in favor of trust in the community's "mutual aid."

Deity/God or Ultimate Other

As an independent free church branch of Christianity, Anabaptists are monotheistic. Most Mennonites have a classical Trinitarian understanding of God as Father, Son, and Holy Spirit. God is deeply concerned with each individual life, inviting each person to a life of Christian discipleship within the church community. Individual and corporate prayer, meditation, and singing are typical means of communicating with God. All Mennonites would also say that God often speaks to us through the insight or wisdom of others and through the words and stories of Christian Scripture.

Views on Health and Well-Being

Health and well-being must be understood in relationship to the kingdom of God in several respects. In the ministries of Jesus and the early church, restoration of physical health from illness or disability was seen as a sign of God's present and coming kingdom. God cares about our physical and mental well-being, and the restoration of such well-being is a sign that God's kingdom is operative in the world. Health and well-being also concerns being restored to proper relationship with God and others. Restored relationships that embody trust, love, patience, generosity, and justice are hallmarks simultaneously of God's kingdom and human well-being.

Physical health should not become an idol sought for its own sake or sought primarily to avoid suffering or to maximize our years on earth. Instead, health is largely valued because it allows us to love God and serve our neighbor. Because our lives are given to us as gifts to be used for God's service, Anabaptist-descended groups have a sense of stewardship about their physical and mental health. Our lives are not our own; they are entrusted to us for God's service. Thus, we should care for our physical and mental well-being (e.g., exercise, consume food or alcohol in moderation, refrain from smoking, maintain prayerful lives) not so much for one's own sake, but for the sake of service to God and neighbor. Because God's kingdom is concerned with human flourishing in the context of re-stored relationships, health and well-being must be conceived in broad, inclusive terms. Thus, for example, fair distribution of wealth, access to clean water and clean air, the elimination of barriers to social participation for those with physical or mental challenges, and so on, are components of health and well-being. Lastly, Anabaptist-descended groups accept the reciprocal responsibility of members within the community to care for each other's emotional, social, spiritual, material, and physical needs. In other words, the components of health and well-being are profoundly social. Not only is health first defined by restored relationships, but those relationships then provide the context for the full range of components of human health and well-being.

Explanations for Disease and Illness

The dominant explanation for illness and disease among Mennonite-related groups is the power of sin—both personal and systemic. Suffering and illness can be the result of personal sin. The disease is not God's punishment of the individual but the result of inappropriate behavior in a broken world. The disease is more a consequence of having walked away from God than of God's punishment. In such cases of personal sin, the illness or suffering can then become an opportunity to repent and to learn to rest secure in God's forgiveness.

While acknowledging the potential role of personal sin, most Anabaptist-descended groups seldom attribute an individual's illness or suffering to personal sin. Instead, these groups most often attribute illness to sin's systemic and cosmic reach. Mennonite-related groups believe that everything from government and military and economic structures to family systems and religious institutions to the very structure of creation itself has been distorted and made susceptible to the dominion of corruption and death by the power of sin. Given this cosmic sense of sin's power, it is natural for Anabaptist-descended groups to see a direct connection between suffering and sin without attributing culpability to the individual sufferers.

This theological account of illness also affirms that illness is a function of viruses, bacteria, genetic mutations, pollution, malnutrition, and so on.

The Nature of Suffering and How to Address It

The meaning associated with suffering depends on its type or cause. Suffering that is the result of discipleship is seen as sharing in the sufferings of Jesus and a participation in Christ's overcoming sin's power in the world (e.g., suffering that comes as a consequence of nonviolently standing for justice or refusing to repay evil with evil). Suffering that is not a result of discipleship is seen as a sign of sin's continuing power in the world and a reminder that we await the full realization of God's kingdom. With all types of suffering, Anabaptist-descended groups have a deep sense that God through Christ understands the nature of human frailty, illness, pain, and loss and that God offers to be intimately present with us in the midst of suffering. In all suffering, one can strive to trust the sufficiency of God's grace and the love of the believing community (whose love can be a sign of God's own presence and a taste of God's already-present-but-also-still-coming kingdom). In many cases of suffering, Mennonites also see an opportunity to grow in certain virtues; patience and humility are often mentioned in this context, although additional virtues such as courage are also clearly relevant.

Death, Dying, and Afterlife

Many Mennonites believe that persons enter into God's presence immediately upon death. Other Mennonites, and the official positions of Mennonite Church USA and Mennonite Church Canada, emphasize a future resurrection of the dead, God's victory over sin and evil, and the complete coming of God's kingdom. In both cases, there is confidence that God finally overcomes pain, suffering, corruption, and death itself. This confidence means that death is not the greatest evil or one to be avoided at all costs. While God's love and final victory provide great comfort and courage, all Anabaptist-descended groups also have some account of God's final judgment: some choose by conviction or practice to be separated from the love of God.

Quick and Condensed Definitions of Terms

Discipleship—Christian faith is about following Jesus in the company of the church in all aspects of life, even to the point of death.

Mutual aid—Anabaptist-descended groups believe that we are called to bear each other's emotional, spiritual, physical, and economic needs. The most dramatic example of this conviction is the Amish barn raising, but this conviction also involves nearly every aspect of life, including medical care and medical bills.

"Discernment" and *"Binding and Loosing"*—When becoming a member of a Mennonite-related church, believers commit themselves to give and receive counsel within the faith community on important matters of doctrine and conduct. Such decision making is most often referred to as discernment, but might be referred to as "binding and loosing," especially when involving a transgression or offering release to someone from repented sin.

God's kingdom—Concerns God's healing and redeeming rule in heaven and on earth; is both a personal and social–political reality. With Jesus and the gift of the Spirit, that kingdom is already operative in the world, but we await the complete manifestation of that kingdom in God's own timing.

Prayer

Prayer is attending to God: talking with God, listening for God's voice, confessing before God, petitioning for others to God. The assumption is that all of life should be prayer filled and prayer directed. Prayer is both individual and corporate. In many church communities, communal prayers for specific individuals suffering from illness are a regular part of gathered worship.

Religious Calendar

In most Mennonite-related communities, at least some attention is given to the Advent through Pentecost cycle of the Christian liturgical year. Church communities often gather on Maundy Thursday and/or Good Friday to share communion. In some communities, Pentecost remains an important day for baptisms. In many conservative Mennonite and Old Order Amish communities, Ascension Day is observed with church services and other social gatherings.

Health-Promoting Practices

Use of tobacco is rare. In most groups, such practices would be explicitly proscribed and frowned upon as poor stewardship. There is limited consensus regarding alcohol. Some would view any consumption of alcohol as sinful, but most groups accept moderate drinking but proscribe any type of heavy drinking or drunkenness. Food plays a major role in the gathered life of many communities. Unfortunately, the food is often high in calories, fat, sugar, and salt.

Healing Rituals

Besides simple visitation and prayers, a patient in an Anabaptist-descended tradition is most likely to request communion and/or anointing with oil. Since communion is understood to be an act of communal remembrance, confession, and reconciliation, it is important to contact the pastor or other leader from the patient's own community if at all possible. While contacting those leaders is also advisable for anointing, many Mennonites would be open to receiving an anointing from the hospital chaplain or Christian clergy if their own leaders are unavailable. This openness is not true, however, for all Anabaptist-descended groups. Anointing nearly always should also include a few close family and friends or fellow church members. Some are open to communion officiated by someone outside their tradition, but this would not be the norm.

Other Unique Religious Beliefs, Rites, and Practices Related to Health or Illness

None.

Unique Religious Beliefs, Rites, and Practices Related to Birthing

Many Amish utilize a midwife (sometimes not licensed by the state) to deliver their children at home or in special birthing centers. The reasons for this common practice are tied to the costs and distance of hospital births, as well as convictions about simplicity.

Unique Religious Beliefs, Rites, or Practices Related to Childrearing

Anabaptists do not baptize infants or young children. If infants or children die too young to make an "adult" decision to follow Christ, they are believed to rest secure in God's grace. Dedication of babies is observed in some less conservative Mennonite congregations with a reminder to the congregants of their responsibility in nurturing the child.

Unique Beliefs, Practices, and Rituals Surrounding Dying, Death, and Bereavement

Most groups have funeral services that are similar to other Protestants. If the person lived a life of love and generosity toward others, the worship service is often marked by a sense of celebration (amidst the grief) of a life well lived in service to God and others. Nearly all funerals will be followed by a fellowship meal, and most will have an open time for sharing of stories about the deceased.

The Amish are distinct in that they typically will keep the deceased body at home until the funeral and internment. Usually, family and community members stay with the body 24 hours a day, and community visitation happens over a period of several days.

Role of Religious Community (Persons or Organizations) During Health Challenges

Most Anabaptist-descended groups meet at least weekly for religious instruction and worship, although most Amish meet every other week. Most groups have designated church buildings or worship space, although most Amish meet in homes. Nearly all services include the reading of Scripture, corporate prayer, and singing. Sharing of communion is less frequent.

In some congregations or communities, individuals might be charged or commissioned with the task of supporting members with health challenges, but such roles are not standardized. It is assumed that members of the congregation will also visit the sick and needy. It is equally assumed that they will provide various forms of comfort care (e.g., bringing meals to the family, providing respite care). The mechanism for coordinating such care is informal, yet typically efficient. In some congregations, coordination is through the deacons or "nurse in the congregation," or "congregational care coordinator."

Role of Clergy During Health Challenges

Ordained clergy, as well as other church leaders, will pray for the ill, especially during hospital or home visits. The visit typically includes informal conversation, scripture, and prayer. It may also include communion or anointing with oil. There is no special efficacy attributed to the prayers of church leaders. It is assumed that all members of the community will hold each other in prayer. However, the prayerful presence of the ordained pastor does seem to symbolize the gathered presence of the church community in a way that is often not true when other church members visit.

Unique Religious Aspects of Family Involvement

Potentially unique is the extent of church involvement in making medical decisions. Commitment to community and an understanding of shared discernment means that all Anabaptist-descended groups are open to the counsel of "brothers" and "sisters" from the community. This shared discernment can be particularly noticeable to nurses dealing with Amish patients. Indeed, what may look like an abrogation of the patient's autonomy to the nurse often fits well with the patient's overall, life-long commitments to the community's life.

Nursing Implications Unique to This Religious Tradition

- Mennonite-related groups believe that life is a gift and that we are entrusted as caretakers of God's good creation. This conviction means an obligation to take care of one's own body through practices such as regular exercise, daily prayer, and moderation in diet. The conviction also means an obligation not to overutilize medical resources so that there are resources for others. Thus, Mennonite-related groups will sometimes reject costly therapy and life-sustaining treatment even when the individual or community can afford them or the treatment would be covered by insurance. Such treatment can be rejected as "poor stewardship," the misuse of God's resources.

- The prayer of the sick may be more of lament and a focus on God's presence, rather than a rumination about "why?" or "why me?"

- Access to Christian Scripture and as much freedom for visitation from family and congregation members are key. New International Version (NIV) and New Revised Standard Version (NRSV) are commonly read translations of the Bible; more conservative believers may prefer King James Version (KJV), and many Amish read in German. In some cases, it is possible to request that recordings of the weekly service be shared with the patient. (This recommendation would not apply to the Old Order Amish who do not use electricity.)

- Congregations typically have remarkably strong informal care coordinators who can mobilize resources for patients and their families. Denominational organizations may also offer support. A full listing of organizations that provide health-related services (including developmental disability services, mental health services, and retirement and nursing home care) can be found at: http://www.mhsonline.org/php/directory/directory.search.php. A church-wide organization to help congregations and families with members who have disabilities is the Anabaptist Disabilities Network: http://www.adnetonline.org/.

- Respect that health care decision making may involve the input of church and family members. The faith community is especially integral to the life of Anabaptist-descended groups.

FOR MORE INFORMATION

Visit Mennonite Church USA at http://www.mennoniteusa.org/, Third Way Café at http://www.thirdway.com/, Mennonite World Conference at http://www. mwc-cmm.org/, or Mennonite Healthcare Fellowship at http://mennhealth. org/.

Anglicans and Episcopalians

CONTRIBUTOR: *The Reverend David T. Gortner, MA, MDiv, PhD*

NURSE REVIEWER: *The Reverend Faye Davenport, RN, BA, BTh, MN, MEd*

Theology and Social History

The Episcopal Church, born out of the Church of England, is part of the Anglican Communion that spread worldwide during the period of the British Empire, through settlements, trade, and mission. In the 1500s, when King Henry VIII dissolved the English Church's ties with the pope in Rome, closed the monasteries and redistributed their lands, allowed English responses and prayers in public worship, and set an English translation of the Bible in every church, he acted on a long-standing tension between church and state on matters of authority. Embattled years of tension that followed between Catholics and Protestants were brought to resolution under Queen Elizabeth I and the English Parliament, when the Church of England sought to establish a form of common Christian worship and leadership that was responsive to both Catholic and Protestant Christian perspectives.

The Anglican Church was among the strongest denominations in Colonial America, but it began to diminish after the breakaway of Methodists and during the Revolution. Following the American Revolution, the Episcopal Church constituted itself in 1787 out of Anglican churches. It published its own Book of Common Prayer (BCP) adapted for the emerging new culture and nation of the United States. From its birth through to the middle of the 20th century, the Episcopal Church was clearly associated with social positions of power, influence, and prestige. Over time, the Church has sought to correct this imbalance and to broaden its membership across social classes and ethnic communities. There are currently just over 2 million members of the Episcopal Church in the United States, as well as member churches in Europe, Haiti, and several other Caribbean nations, Ecuador, Colombia, Venezuela, and Taiwan.

A love of worship and a commitment to worship in the common language of the people, a desire to chart a spacious "Middle Way" that is at once both Catholic and Reformed, and a resistance to foreign church authority all are part of the spirit that shapes the Anglican Churches worldwide and the Episcopal Church (Anglican/Episcopal [A/E]). Anglicans are bound together by the Bible, by the heritage of the BCP (translated and adapted to different languages and cultures), by broadly common understandings of baptism and holy communion, and by a common structure of church leadership and Christian discipleship. Anglicans are not bound together by an enforced uniformity, a centralized worldwide ruling hierarchy, or a set of rules or beliefs understood as unique only to Anglicans. The spirit of unity in the worldwide Anglican Communion is through a commitment to relationship and common good, respectful of the unique challenges in each country and region of the world.

There have been a few schisms and new denominations from the Episcopal Church. These include the Reformed Episcopal Church (begun in 1874), the Charismatic Episcopal Church (1992), and the various churches and dioceses that have broken ties with the Episcopal Church and aligned themselves with Anglican Churches in Africa or South America (particularly following the Episcopal Church's ordination of women in the 1970s and more recently in the open recognition of gay and lesbian couples and the consecration of gay and lesbian bishops in committed life partnerships). The Episcopal Church's decisions, along with those of other Anglican churches in other countries, have stirred tensions in the Anglican Communion and challenged its unity. But despite these challenges and tensions that arise in different times and places, the Episcopal Church and its Anglican associates around the world remain absolutely committed to following Jesus Christ and to serving people in all places on earth.

Deity/God or Ultimate Other

As Christians, A/Es believe in one God. In creeds and in the prayers of public worship, God is known and adored as Triune or Three in One. A/Es know and experience this one God as Father (Creator and Source of all being), as Son (Redeemer, God known in Jesus Christ), and Holy Spirit (Sustainer of life). God is almighty and above all creation, and yet intimately present to and with all beings. A/Es believe in and affirm a God who is always present, who does not withdraw from creation but has embraced creation even to the point of even taking on human nature in Jesus Christ. Communication with God is always possible, through the mundane as well as the sacred—because, through Christ and through the Holy Spirit, God is present in all things and in all people. A/Es believe that God created human beings in God's own image, that this image has not been erased or completely distorted by sin (i.e., deliberate disobedience of God's will), and that this image is fully restored through the redeeming life, death, and resurrection of Jesus Christ. Episcopalians promise at their baptism to "seek and serve Christ in each person"—to honor the presence of the Holy in all others. This belief and promise arises out of encounter with God in communal and individual prayer, receiving of the sacraments, hearing and reading the scriptures, conversation/ fellowship with others, service, quiet reflection. Episcopalians also seek and find God in the ordinary stuff of daily life: in family, friends, and strangers;

in food and drink; in work, school, rest, and play; in service, sickness, and celebration.

Views on Health and Well-Being

Health and well-being, like life itself, are gifts and graces of God. They are not rewards for good behavior, yet there are clear physical and psychological consequences of certain behavioral choices. Likewise, sickness is not understood as a direct result of sin or personal wrongdoing. Sickness can simply result from the nature of being in the world. It can also be an unfortunate consequence of being harmed or sinned against by others. Most importantly, sickness and death are not the final destinies of human beings. Resurrection, judgment, and a final destiny awaits each person at the return of Christ, the end of history as currently experienced, and the beginning of a "new heaven and new earth."

Explanations for Disease and Illness

Jesus was asked by his disciples to explain a man's blindness: Was it because of personal or family sin? Jesus responded that it was because of neither and that God's glory would be revealed through his sickness. As Christians, A/Es do not view disease and illness as a direct result of sin. However, disease and illness often bring times of reflection on life and its failures, and people often wonder if they are to blame for what has happened to them. Because of this, and in the case of situations when illness is linked to choices made in someone's life, the rite of "Ministration to the Sick" includes confession of sin. In all circumstances of life, the distortions of sin and the grace of God may be found.

The Nature of Suffering and How to Address It

Suffering is not punishment or a sign of God's disfavor. Suffering and blessing come to the just and the unjust alike in this life. However, some forms of suffering result from choices people make, and some forms of suffering are the unfortunate consequence of choices other people make. A/Es do not generally believe that God inflicts suffering in order to teach people lessons. Nonetheless, suffering can be instructive; it can teach us about our limitations and unrecognized strengths and weaknesses. Suffering also can bring people closer to God and more in touch with their own mortality and dependency on God and other people. In this sense, suffering, like any other ordinary reality in human life, is something that may be sanctified by God and infused as a source of unexpected grace.

Death, Dying, and Afterlife

Death is a natural part of the life cycle and of creation. Death is sad for those still living; mourning and bereavement are also natural, a part of God's creation. The dead rest in the Lord until the final day of resurrection and judgment. What this time of "resting in the Lord" is like, no mortal knows. Some conceive of it as something like heaven or hell, others as "soul sleep." Indeed, beliefs vary about the nature of the new life that awaits people after death. Beliefs range from a final awaited day of resurrection of the whole person, to a more commonly held belief in an afterlife of souls who are with God awaiting the final day of resurrection of the body. Hell, heaven, and final judgment are part of the Church's tradition, but among many A/Es, there is a generous sense of God's benevolence and Christ's death being "not for our sins only, but for the sins of the whole world."

The A/E faith and recognition of the mystery of God's redeeming work at the time of death is exemplified in the following prayer offered with people gathered at the time of someone's death: "Into your hands, O merciful Savior, we commend your servant [name]. Acknowledge, we humbly beseech you, a sheep of your own fold, a lamb of your own flock, a sinner of your own redeeming. Receive him/her into the arms of your mercy, into the blessed rest of everlasting peace, and into the glorious company of the saints in light. Amen" (BCP, p. 465). A/Es stress respectful care of the body after death, and it is typical for families to work with a priest to plan a funeral.

Quick and Condensed Definitions of Terms

Holy Eucharist—Known in other Christian circles as Holy Communion or the Lord's Supper. To receive Holy Eucharist is to be fed and nourished directly by Christ and to be made one with Christ and other Christians.

Priest, Deacon, Bishop—Titles of ordained ministers in the Church. A priest may be referred to as Pastor, Reverend, Father, or Mother. Priests are the ministers of sacraments in the Church. Deacons are ordained ministers of service and public witness, who often serve as pastoral caregivers. Bishops are regional leaders of the Church.

Rector, Vicar, Chaplain—These are titles for priests that serve as senior or solo pastors of congregations, or as pastors serving institutions.

Anointing (or unction), laying on of hands—Ways in which a priest, bishop, or appointed pastoral minister may pray with someone who is sick or dying. Anointing with oil is considered a sacramental rite of healing.

Prayer

For A/Es, prayer is both individual and corporate. It is communication and communion with God. It may include words as well as silence. There are many forms of prayer, including praise and thanksgiving, petitions and requests, and contemplation. Clergy and laypeople alike pray for one another privately and during corporate worship. Prayers are said with and around someone who is ill, as requested. A/Es are most at ease with written or memorized prayers (including the Psalms from scripture) and are generally comfortable with visits from clergy or lay pastoral visitors. As a part of prayer, a priest may lay hands upon someone who is ill or anoint the person with a small bit of blessed oil.

Daily prayer is encouraged of all members, in sickness and health. Many A/Es pray the Daily Offices of Morning Prayer and Evening Prayer, and read a scripture assigned for each day. These rites, and simpler devotional rites for various times of the day, are found in the BCP. All Episcopalians know the Lord's Prayer.

Religious Calendar

Like other liturgical Western churches (e.g., Lutherans, Roman Catholics), A/Es follow a religious calendar. The seasons of the year (beginning in December) are Advent, Christmas, Epiphany, Lent, Eastertide, and Pentecost. These seasons mark the story of the faith and of God's redeeming work. Christmas and Easter are the principal days, but there are other important principal "Feast Days" in the Church: Epiphany (which concludes the 12 days of Christmas), Pentecost, All Saints Day, and Trinity Sunday. Other important days and seasons include Ash Wednesday (which marks the beginning of Lent—the 46 days prior to Easter), Palm Sunday, and all of Holy Week immediately before Easter, and the Sunday after Thanksgiving, which usually marks the beginning of the season of Advent. There are also various days throughout the year that mark the lives of saints of the Church. These days will be more or less meaningful to individuals depending upon their level of devotion, immersion, and/or history in the A/E Church.

Health-Promoting Practices

Episcopalians are highly flexible and permissive when it comes to dietary matters. A/Es are encouraged, but not commanded, to fast or give up some foods, or to simplify their diets, during Lent. Some A/Es (more on the Catholic end of the spectrum) keep a partial or total fast on Fridays throughout the year.

Healing Rituals

A/E members vary widely in their desire for healing rituals. For those who desire rituals of healing, such rituals may include prayer with family or friends, saying the Lord's Prayer, receiving the laying on of hands or anointing with oil by a priest or designated pastoral care provider ("Ministration of the Sick"), or receiving the Holy Eucharist.

Other Unique Religious Beliefs, Rites, and Practices Related to Health or Illness

Beliefs, rites, and practices related to health and illness are similar to those for Roman Catholics, mainline Protestants, and many evangelical Protestants. There are some, but not many, charismatic Episcopalians whose prayer practices and beliefs around illness might resemble those of Pentecostals.

Unique Religious Beliefs, Rites, and Practices Related to Birthing

There are no mandated religious practices regarding the birth process. Male circumcision may or may not be requested by parents. Practices will vary more by culture, family background, and personal desires of parents. There are prayers that may be said at the birth of a child, by family members, friends, or clergy (see "Liturgies and prayers related to childbearing, childbirth, and loss").

Unique Religious Beliefs, Rites, or Practices Related to Childrearing

Baptism is the sacrament of new birth in Christ, the sure sign of the grace of salvation offered by God. In Holy Baptism, "the promises of the forgiveness of sin, and of our adoption to be the sons of God by the Holy Ghost, are visibly signed and sealed" (BCP, p. 873). Children and babies may be baptized, and parents make promises on behalf of their children. "The bond which God establishes in Baptism is indissoluble" (BCP, p. 298). Priests and bishops are the sacramental ministers who administer baptism. However, any baptized Christian may administer baptism to another person in life-threatening emergencies, including infants not expected to live. It is pastorally acceptable, but not necessary, to baptize infants (including those stillborn or dead). A/Es believe that babies who do not survive to childhood are held in the eternal embrace of God.

Children are encouraged, but not always required, to participate in religious services, to say prayers at bedtime, and to learn the core stories and teachings of the Bible. Parents vary widely in their practices of religious education with their children. Children "coming of age" were traditionally expected to complete instruction and preparation for the rite of Confirmation. This rite is not always used in current church practices, and other rites are being used to mark transition to adulthood and adult faith.

Unique Beliefs, Practices, and Rituals Surrounding Dying, Death, and Bereavement

A/Es do not have particularly distinctive practices around dying, death, and bereavement. Traditions are informed by both Catholic and Protestant perspectives and practices. Prayers such as the following over the dying are powerful expressions of faith, but are not required:

> Depart, O Christian soul, out of this world; in the Name of God the Father Almighty who created you; in the Name of Jesus Christ who redeemed you; in the Name of the Holy Spirit who sanctifies you. May your rest be this day in peace, and your dwelling place in the Paradise of God. (BCP, p. 464)

Death customs are adaptable to the various cultures in which A/Es live. Funerals are more typical than memorial services and are celebrations of the promise of resurrection and often include the Holy Eucharist. There are no prescribed periods of bereavement.

Role of Religious Community (Persons or Organizations) During Health Challenges

A/Es meet every Sunday and on major holy days for worship, primarily, but also for Christian instruction. Holy Eucharist (communion) is the central act of worship, devotion, and connection with God. At each gathering for worship, Episcopalians offer praise to God, listen to scripture, pray, and seek God's blessing and strengthening. Worship conforms to the BCP and its supplements.

Congregations include the sick and shut-in in their prayers at these services. Following any celebration of the Holy Eucharist, a congregation may send out a visitor (ordained or lay) with reserved sacrament to extend this celebration to the sick. This Eucharistic Visitor will often bring a worship bulletin, follow the same prayers and readings, review key points from the sermon, and share communion with the ill person.

Many churches have Stephen's Ministers who are laypersons providing an hour of care per week to members who are physically or emotionally hurting. These lay caregivers receive structured training and supervision. Some parishes have parish nurses. Many have congregational lay pastoral teams that work with priests and deacons to provide care on behalf of the congregation.

Role of Clergy During Health Challenges

Priests, deacons, and lay pastoral visitors are expected to visit and tend the sick. Care for the sick is an expectation a parish will have of its clergy.

Unique Religious Aspects of Family Involvement

Family members are involved in ways similar to other Catholic and Protestant families with loved ones who are ill.

Nursing Implications Unique to This Religious Tradition

- A nurse can ask A/E patients if they would like to receive communion on a Sunday and if they belong to a parish that can send a Eucharistic Visitor. If the patient is not connected to a church in the area, a priest or Eucharistic Visitor can still be requested to bring communion from a local parish.

- To arrange other healing rituals or a pastoral visit, the nurse ought to work with the institution's chaplains. If there are no formal spiritual carers, then the nurse can contact the local A/E parish (ideally, the parish where the patient attends).

- Many A/Es will observe a partial fast during the Lenten season. Often, this means the individual chooses to refrain from eating certain foods (e.g., chocolate, sweets, meat).

FOR MORE INFORMATION

The Episcopal Church. (1979). *Book of common prayer.* Oxford, UK: Oxford University Press.

The Episcopal Church. (2010). *Enriching our worship 5: Liturgies and prayers related to childbearing, childbirth, and loss.* New York, NY: Church Publishing.

The Episcopal Church. (2005). *Ministry with the sick.* New York, NY: Church Publishing.

Griswold, F. T. (2009). *Praying our days: A guide and companion.* New York, NY: Morehouse.

Hein, D., & Shattuck, G. H., Jr. (2005). *The Episcopalians.* New York, NY: Church Publishing.

Schmidt, R. H. (2002). *Glorious companions: Five centuries of Anglican spirituality.* Grand Rapids, MI: Eerdmans.

10 Atheists

CONTRIBUTOR: *David Silverman*
NURSE REVIEWER: *Caz Hales, BNurs (Hons), PG Dip, RN*

Theology and Social History

Atheism is probably the oldest philosophy in the world and likely outdates all religions. Religion was invented by humans to answer the Grand Questions in a manner that atheism could not and still cannot. Atheists, however, believe these answers are fictional. By classical definition, atheists deny the existence of any gods. In contemporary society, persons who reject religion and theism may label themselves variously as atheists, freethinkers, secular humanists, or another term (see "Quick and Condensed Definitions of Terms").

Atheists love for their beliefs to be respected and acknowledged, especially given atheists rarely do get such respect. Currently, atheists are the most disliked group of people in the United States. Atheists are a people against whom it is still politically correct to discriminate; they feel such discrimination regularly. However, atheists are also the fastest growing segment in all 50 states, so are experiencing the tide of change. American Atheists, founded by Madalyn Murray O'Hair in 1963, has been a leader of this change. Pew Research Center findings indicate that atheists are more educated than theists, highly intelligent, and know a lot about religion.

Deity/God or Ultimate Other

Atheists agree there are no deities, no ghosts, no devils of any kind.

Views on Health and Well-Being

To be healthy means to be free of disease, both mental and physical. There is nothing "spiritual"; therefore, the notion of spiritual health is foreign and offensive. Atheists would accept definitions of health that are void of the notion of spiritual well-being.

Explanations for Disease and Illness

Atheists accept scientific and medically supported explanations for the causes of disease. They would, of course, reject that there is any supernatural influence on any disease process.

The Nature of Suffering and How to Address It

Suffering is terrible and real. It happens without regard to how good or bad a person is or has been. It is a natural result of natural events, and it should be addressed with medicines. However, it should be noted that laughter and the comfort of loved ones do have psychological effects that are very real and should not be ignored.

Death, Dying, and Afterlife

Death is the end of life. It happens to every living thing in the universe. It is nonexistence. Facing death is difficult, and this is the very reason religion and gods were invented in the first place. An atheist facing death is probably scared but will not be comforted at all by religion or religious intrusion.

There is no afterlife, no Grand Plan. Heaven is what we make of our life on earth, for the brief period we exist.

Quick and Condensed Definitions of Terms

Atheist—Someone who does not believe in any god. Many atheists do not like the label "atheist," so will use one of the following terms:

Agnostic—Often misused to mean someone who is unsure but actually means someone who understands that the universe is not understandable. Agnostics should be treated as atheists.

Secular Humanist—Atheist with a set of strong moral and ethical values that provide meaning and direction in life, like altruism and benevolence; most likely to attend monthly meetings with others who share their worldview.

Ethical Culturist—Very like a humanist, but more bookish; Ethical Culture is considered a nontheistic religion by the U.S. government.

Rationalist or Secularist—Treat as atheist.

Skeptic—Not specifically atheist; highly scientific in nature; treat as atheist.

Cultural Jew—An atheist of Jewish descent. Many Cultural Jews regard Judaism as a nationality, separable from belief in God.

Prayer

Given there is no god, atheists do not pray.

Religious Calendar

Atheists observe no holy days. Christmas is seen as a religious holiday. Although its religious meanings are rejected, it is enjoyed by many atheists—particularly those raised in Christian homes, as a cultural holiday. Indeed, most employers and schools in Christian-dominated societies plan vacations and days off reflecting the Christian holiday calendar, even though not all are Christians.

Health-Promoting Practices

Empirically supported health practices would be implemented by an atheist (e.g., diet, exercise, laughter, love).

Healing Rituals

None. Atheists will follow medical advice, accepting the best medicine supported by the best research. It should be noted that atheists are skeptics and are not likely to be interested in homeopathic remedies, energy channeling, new-age crystals, and other such "treatments."

Other Unique Religious Beliefs, Rites, and Practices Related to Health or Illness

Not applicable.

Unique Religious Beliefs, Rites, and Practices Related to Birthing

Most atheists are starting to lean away from circumcision, viewing it as a barbaric ritual left over from ancient times. Some still do it, however, so it is important to inquire and offer medical opinion if necessary (supported by science, not tradition).

Unique Religious Beliefs, Rites, or Practices Related to Childrearing

None. Atheists want to do their best to raise a happy and healthy child. Atheists have no notion of a "proper" family; they accept that a family can be formed by partners of any race, gender, or sexual orientation. Although some atheists (e.g., humanists, Ethical Culturalists) create a secular rite of passage (to adulthood) for their children, most do not. This event celebrating a child's accomplishment may occur anytime between the ages of 11 and 16.

Unique Beliefs, Practices, and Rituals Surrounding Dying, Death, and Bereavement

End-of-life practices of atheists reflect, of course, their reality that there are no ghosts, spirits, or afterlife. Thus, it is important for atheists to recognize the purpose, significance, positive personality, and legacy of the dying or deceased person. Atheists find comfort in remembering what the deceased accomplished, even if it was just being a good person, loving parent, or child. It is important to understand that grief is real and profound for an atheist, just as death is real.

Role of Religious Community (Persons or Organizations) During Health Challenges

Atheists often are happy to find other atheists with whom they can converse and share experiences. This typically happens via social media such as internet blogs and chat rooms, which have been a catalyst for the recent trend in increased numbers of atheists. Printed media (e.g., The Freethinker, Secular Nation, and American Atheist Magazine) also allow atheists to communicate with each other. For the most part, social gatherings are not very important to atheists. A few atheists attend monthly meetings at a local Humanist gathering, but this is a minority. For such people (e.g., Secular Humanists and Ethical Culturists), the leader of the meetings is often somewhat influential. Some atheist organizations (e.g., American Atheists) have conventions and, perhaps, a holiday party in the winter.

There are no atheist-sponsored organizations with the purpose of caring for the sick. When atheists are sick, they go to hospitals and get scientifically tested health care.

Role of Clergy During Health Challenges

Not applicable.

Unique Religious Aspects of Family Involvement

Atheists may be especially dependent on family and friends for support, given the absence of clergy or religious community for support. A serious family issue for atheist patients, however, emerges when religious family members wish to convert their loved one. It is insulting and demoralizing when a preaching family member overtly or covertly attempts to produce a deathbed (or sickbed) conversion. Such behavior reflects the proselytizing family member's need, not the needs of the sick or dying atheist.

Nursing Implications Unique to This Religious Tradition

- Because atheists love to meet fellow atheists and not feel alone in their beliefs, nurses who are atheists can bring particular comfort to an atheist patient if they disclose this shared perspective.

- Trying to create a deathbed (or sickbed) conversion is the worst thing to do to an atheist. Doing so would be adding insult to injury. Instead, offer congratulations on successes during life or recognize the impact the patient has made on the society and country.

- Grief for an atheist is a very real, relevant part of life. Support a positive meaning of that life by allowing atheists to talk about their kids, grandkids, accomplishments, and other legacies. Do not offer faith-based statements of comfort as these are inappropriate and rude to an atheist.

- Never offer prayer to an atheist, and do not say someone is praying for the patient (e.g., "I'll be keeping you in my prayers"). Atheists are very proud, and sometimes conceited, about their atheism. Offering any kind of prayer is insulting and degrading.

- Nurses in religious hospitals would do well to offer to remove religious icons in the atheist patient's room. Indeed, they should just do it without asking.

- Given that the atheist worldview rejects the existence of a spiritual reality or any gods, nurses will do well to avoid any reference to such when caring for an atheist patient. "Spiritual" well-being is not an applicable concept in nursing care for atheists.

- When a proselytizing family member causes distress for an atheist patient, nurses can support the patient by clarifying who they desire to have visit and helping the family to support these wishes. A patient so traumatized may also benefit from the nurse's empathic listening to debrief. The nurse may also support the dejected proselytizer by listening empathically so insight can be gained or make a referral to a spiritual care expert.

FOR MORE INFORMATION

Visit www.atheists.org

Dawkins, R. (2008). *The god delusion*. New York, NY: Houghton Mifflin.

Harris, S. (2006). *Letter to a Christian nation*. New York, NY: Knopf.

Ingersoll, R. G. (1900). *Complete lectures of Col. R. G. Ingersoll*. Whitefish, MT: Kessinger.

Baptists

CONTRIBUTOR: *The Reverend Peter Yuichi Clark, PhD*
NURSE REVIEWER: *Christina Miller, MS, MDiv, MA, RN*

Theology and Social History

Baptists evolved as a distinct stream in Protestant Christianity during the early 1600s, mainly in reaction to the clerical structure of the Church of England, which insisted that all British subjects belong to an Anglican parish near their residence. By contrast, Baptists asserted that church membership should be voluntary and that individuals have the capacity and free will to interpret the Bible and follow their own consciences. The belief that baptism should reflect a believer's choice rather than be administered in infancy is indicated in the name "Baptists." Throughout their history, Baptists have been strong advocates for the principles of religious liberty and the separation of church and state in citizens' lives.

Currently, there are 46 to 100 million Baptists worldwide and over 35 million in the United States who organize themselves primarily at the local congregational level, determining their own polity and doctrinal affirmations. (The lack of a centralized organizing structure, which is characteristic of Baptist life, makes exact figures somewhat difficult.) However, many Baptist churches are also affiliated with larger national denominations. In the United States, the four best known bodies are the evangelically oriented Southern Baptist Convention (16.2 million members), the mainline American Baptist Churches USA (1.3 million members), and two historically African American organizations (the National Baptist Convention USA [8 million members] and the Progressive National Baptist Convention [2.5 million members]).

Deity/God or Ultimate Other

Like many Protestant Christians, Baptists believe in a Trinitarian God who is customarily known as Father, Son, and Holy Spirit. Because of God's redeeming compassion, human beings can enjoy a personal relationship with God. The key to beginning such a relationship is through explicitly admitting that one needs God's grace in one's life, confessing Jesus of Nazareth as God's Son, and accepting His living presence in one's life as Lord and Savior—what Baptists term "being saved" or "born again." Scripture reading, frequent prayer, and regular interaction with other believers are deemed vital to sustaining this divine–human relationship.

Views on Health and Well-Being

Health and well-being are desirable. Many Baptists hear the Apostle Paul's teaching that "your body is a temple of the Holy Spirit within you" (I Corinthians 6:19) as a call to live as healthfully as possible. Physical health, however, is subordinate to the state of one's spiritual health.

Explanations for Disease and Illness

Baptists vary greatly in their understanding of the meaning one can attribute to disease and illness. A teaching that many Baptists find instructive appears in the *Gospel of John*, when Jesus is asked why a man was born blind: "Neither this man nor his parents sinned," Jesus replies; "he was born blind so that God's works might be revealed in him" (9:3 New Revised Standard Version [NRSV]). Hence, most Baptists do not attach a moral valuation to illness; yet some might interpret illness as an opportunity to deepen one's faith through endurance, prayer, and devotion to God.

The Nature of Suffering and How to Address It

Because of Baptist roots in Calvinist teachings, there is a doctrinal thread that views suffering as an inevitable consequence of the adverse effect of human sinful behavior on the natural world over the centuries. While most Baptists would not equate the amount of suffering any given individual is experiencing with a specific lack of virtue in that person's life (see above), some do hold that if one is free from doubt and prays fervently for a miraculous healing, God will grant the recovery one seeks. Occasionally, Baptist families of a patient receiving artificial life support measures will ask hospital staff to prolong those treatments to allow God the time to create such a miracle.

Death, Dying, and Afterlife

Death is the end of a person's temporal existence, but there is an essence to human life that transcends death, normally called the soul or spirit. Because there is no central doctrinal authority for Baptists, there is a wide range of interpretations about what happens after death. Some Baptists believe in heaven and hell, and hence, the disposition of a person's soul after death will depend on whether that person had confessed faith in Christ during her or his life. If that person was "saved," then she or he is assured of an everlasting life with God in heaven. Consequently, some families of Baptist patients might become adamant about ensuring the salvation of their loved ones before death, sometimes hoping that they will regain consciousness long enough to make a profession of faith. Other Baptists do not hold as firmly to the concept of hell and would affirm that ultimately God's mercy and judgment are beyond human understanding, so there can be no certainty about the state of any person's postmortem destiny. For those Baptists, an assurance of God's presence and unfailing love in all circumstances may yield a real sense of comfort.

Quick and Condensed Definitions of Terms

"Being saved" or *"born again"*—see definition in section on Deity/God or Ultimate Other.

Communion or *Lord's Supper*—a symbolic re-enactment of Jesus' last meal with his disciples.

Prayer

Prayer is a vital component of one's relationship with God. Because Baptists assert that all believers have equal access to God, prayer is practiced both by individuals and in congregational settings. Most Baptists learn to pray extemporaneously—that is, without utilizing a prayer book or missal. Baptists also believe in intercessory prayer, in which they beseech God's help for those around them who are ill or suffering. In addition to these spontaneous prayers, Baptists also rely on familiar biblical passages such as the Lord's Prayer and the 23rd Psalm.

Religious Calendar

Regular weekly worship services on Sundays are very important to most Baptists. Some Baptists observe the Christian liturgical calendar (e.g., Advent, Christmas, Lent, Holy Week, Easter, Pentecost, etc.), while others recognize Christmas Day and Easter Sunday as the most important holy days. The rituals marking these holy days will vary greatly based on individual churches' practice.

Health-Promoting Practices

Because of the Apostle Paul's teaching about our physical bodies as temples (see above), Baptists traditionally have refrained from alcohol and tobacco. Controlled substances would be discouraged and their use limited to medically prescribed and supervised use. Some Baptists hold to these practices more strictly than others. There are no other dietary proscriptions.

Healing Rituals

Believers frequently will ask for prayer when ill. Some Baptists will ask for "the laying on of hands" or anointing with oil in conjunction with prayers. There is no uniform practice for this healing ritual. Although ministers and deacons typically do it, there is no prohibition against a layperson doing it.

Other Unique Religious Beliefs, Rites, and Practices Related to Health or Illness

None beyond what has already been mentioned.

Unique Religious Beliefs, Rites, and Practices Related to Birthing

Baptists do not baptize infants. This practice stems from the belief that baptism is a symbol of an individual's intentional decision to become a Christian; a person, therefore, must be of an age and developmental capacity so as to make that conscious choice. Most Baptists would neither discourage nor endorse a specific age. Many Baptist churches will offer a blessing to a baby soon after the family has resumed attending worship services, but there are no mandated rites or practices related to childbirth.

Unique Religious Beliefs, Rites, or Practices Related to Childrearing

Because Baptists believe in the need for all human beings to enjoy an unmediated and direct interaction with God, Baptist families often involve their children in Sunday School (an educational time that usually precedes the worship service), and they encourage their children to profess their faith in Christ as soon as they appear to understand the moral implications of their actions—what is commonly known as "the age of accountability." Teens are also invited to participate in church-based youth group activities throughout their high school years.

Unique Beliefs, Practices, and Rituals Surrounding Dying, Death, and Bereavement

Because Baptists adhere to a belief in individual competency to make decisions, each Baptist is free to decide about organ donation and also about burial or cremation after death. Baptist rituals after death can involve a memorial service, a funeral, a graveside service, or any combination of these options.

Role of Religious Community (Persons or Organizations) During Health Challenges

Baptists usually worship together in churches on Sunday mornings. Some churches also will have Sunday evening and midweek services. Worship services normally include congregational hymns, Bible readings, prayers, a sermon, a collection or offering of money to support the church's charitable works, and frequently an invitation or "altar call" where people are invited to publicly declare their decision to become Christians. At regular intervals in the church calendar—monthly or quarterly—the congregation will observe the Lord's Supper or Communion, and occasionally, new believers will be baptized.

A Baptist patient who is strongly attached to her or his congregation may desire to receive Communion on the Sunday that corresponds to her or his church's regular schedule, if possible. Most Baptist churches assign this responsibility to their pastoral staff and to their deacons (laypersons who have been formally selected to assist in the governance and ministries of the church).

However, a key element in Baptist doctrine is that all people, whether ordained or not, are seen as equal in the eyes of God, and therefore anyone can provide vital ministry to those who need physical assistance or spiritual comfort. Hence, some congregations organize themselves into caregiving teams that mobilize when particular persons or families assigned to them experience crises (like hospitalization) or transitions (welcoming a newborn baby, for example). Members of these teams will cook meals for families, visit ill persons in the hospital or at home, and bring Communion.

Role of Clergy During Health Challenges

Frequently, pastors and deacons will lead prayers on behalf of ill congregation members during regular worship services. It is not uncommon for a minister, a deacon, or several members of the church's leadership team to visit an ill member and offer prayers for his or her recovery.

Unique Religious Aspects of Family Involvement

None.

Nursing Implications Unique to This Religious Tradition

- Baptists consider the Bible to be central in their daily lives and spiritual practice. If a Baptist patient requested someone to read from the Bible, know that Psalms, the Gospel accounts of Jesus' ministry, and the letters attributed to the Apostle Paul (e.g., Romans, Galatians, Ephesians) are most frequently cited.

- Baptists also have an enduring tradition of congregational singing in their worship, so an awareness of hymns, gospel songs, and African American spirituals can be useful in relating to Baptist patients.

- If a nurse is comfortable offering a prayer, in most cases, it would be gratefully received. Nurses and other clinicians should feel free to consult the chaplain or the pastor from a local Baptist church if spiritual needs arise.

FOR MORE INFORMATION

Visit Southern Baptist Convention at http://www.sbc.net/, American Baptist Churches USA at http://www.abc-usa.org/, National Baptist Convention USA at http://www.nationalbaptist.com/, Progressive National Baptist Convention at http://www.pnbc.org/PNBC/Home.html, or Baptist World Alliance at http://www.bwanet.org/

12 Buddhists

CONTRIBUTOR: *Tony Toneatto, PhD, CPsych*
NURSE REVIEWER: *Jessica Ongley, RN*

Theology and Social History

Buddhism is based on the teachings of Siddhartha Gautama (or Shakyamuni Buddha) who lived from 563 to 483 BCE. At the age of 35, following many years of arduous spiritual disciplines and meditation, and as a result of the profound realization of the causes and conditions of suffering and the means by which to eliminate suffering, he came to be called the Buddha, or "the Awakened Mind." After this Enlightenment, Buddha spent the bulk of the rest of his life teaching others how to also awaken their own mind, and he attracted an increasing number of disciples or devotees. From its original home in what is now Nepal, Buddhism spread throughout Asia—especially India, Sri Lanka, Vietnam, Cambodia, Laos, China, Japan, Tibet, Thailand, Burma, and Afghanistan.

Buddhist spiritual life is centered in the community, the teachings of the Buddha and commentaries, and the Buddha himself. Although varying across different Buddhist traditions, Buddhism tends to be nontheistic, focusing on the importance of developing oneself to the best of one's ability. However, most Buddhist temples and religious centers will display statues of the Buddha and other Buddhist saints and divinities to remind oneself of one's spiritual potential. Buddhist practitioners, except for monks and nuns who may dress in traditional robes, shave their heads and follow strict guidelines regarding diet, possessions, and lifestyle, are not distinguished by any specific clothing, food preference, or lifestyle. The temple remains the center of religious teaching and ritual practice and serves as a focal point in preserving, teaching, and applying Buddhist teachings. A distinguishing aspect of Buddhist teaching is the strong encouragement that followers should test and verify for themselves the truth of Buddha teachings rather than to rely on authority, dogma, or belief.

Deity/God or Ultimate Other

While the earliest forms of Buddhism, especially those traditions found in southern Asia were considered to be nontheistic (and generally classified as Theravadin Buddhism), later traditions—especially in Northern Asia, developed extensive pantheons of Buddhist divinities (and are generally classified as Mahayana Buddhism). These deities are believed to assist the practitioner to become enlightened by developing the necessary spiritual qualities needed and to weaken hindrances to self-knowledge. These deities, however, are not considered all-powerful or eternal. A popular development with Buddhism—Vajrayana, or Trantric Buddhism—developed in Tibet about a millennium ago and continues to be popularized today by the Dalai Lama, the titular head of Vajrayana Buddhism.

Views on Health and Well-Being

Buddhists view health as consisting of specific beliefs, attitudes, and practices that are conducive to peace of mind and equanimity. These are expressed through compassion and lovingkindness to all sentient beings, including oneself, other people, as well as the animal kingdom. To achieve this state of health requires that one attain specific insights, especially the clarity that (1) all experiences, things, and phenomena are impermanent; (2) they are incapable of producing true and lasting happiness; and (3) they lack inherent or eternal existence. (These are often called the "three marks of existence.") To the degree that we hold the opposite view, we will continually search for sources of happiness outside of oneself. Thus, one will be prone to disappointment, loss, and all varieties of emotional distress. The Buddha advocated concentration and meditation as well as skillful behavior, speech, livelihood—exemplified in treating others with love and compassion, as the means by which one could realize these specific insights. Success in adopting and integrating these perspectives and actions into our day-to-day life constitutes optimal health.

Explanations for Disease and Illness

Disease and illness are inescapable aspects of the human condition that no one can avoid. The causes of illness are generally explained a naturalistic way that is consistent with modern scientific understandings that emphasize causes and conditions. While some causes and conditions may be outside our direct control (e.g., public health policies, genetics, accidents, disasters), many causes and conditions of disease and illness are within our control. Buddhist teachings specifically identify unskillful lifestyles and behaviors, characterized by disturbances in harmony, balance, moderation, and emotions (excessive eating, intoxication, stress, anger, and the like), as important contributors to illness. Hence, the Buddhist advice of moderation and balance, both mentally and physically, is advocated as an important means by which illness can be reduced.

The Nature of Suffering and How to Address It

The Buddha's first teaching after his Enlightenment concerned suffering and its ubiquity and pervasiveness. The Buddha taught that suffering included not only the agony that is associated with great physical pain but also the subtle suffering of disappointment, loss, and change. In Buddhist teachings, all phenomena have the potential to produce suffering. However, the Buddha also distinguished *pain* (which is generally unavoidable and usually originates from the physical world) from *suffering* (which reflects one's attitudes toward the pain and generally originates from our mind). He also identified the cause of suffering as strong, unremitting need or craving in which we project our needs and desires on the outside world, truly believing that the outside world is the source of authentic happiness. In other words, suffering arises when what *we want* we cannot have, keep, or get, or what *we do not want* will not go away, returns, or persists. To the degree that we resist such vicissitudes of life by persisting in assuming that the world can reliably bring us happiness, to that degree we will experience suffering. To escape suffering, the Buddha advocates a deep, intuitive understanding of the impermanence of all perceived phenomena, the unreliability of the world to genuinely and permanently satisfy us, and the lack of inherent identity or essence of things. Combined with the nurturance of compassion and lovingkindness, ethical behavior (verbally, behaviorally, emotionally), and emotional balance and equanimity, we can minimize suffering and achieve enduring health.

Death, Dying, and Afterlife

The self (consisting of five interdependent and interactive elements: *the physical body, consciousness, cognition–perception, emotion,* and *conditioned habits*) is viewed as an unending process, consisting of the constant arising, abiding, and subsiding of moments of experience linked together by memory and physical continuity. Most Buddhist traditions equate death with the dissolution of these five elements into their elemental components. While the primordial life force and stream of consciousness is believed to persist through rebirth, the consciousness in the reborn person is not identical to that which was in the deceased person. The reborn person is the outcome of a causal continuum of mental events that characterized and comprised the previous life and now continues to be expressed in the reborn life. The specific attributes and characteristics of the reborn person will be causally connected to the quality and nature of their character and behavior of their previous life but cannot be viewed as a continuation of the previous life. Thus, Buddhists are encouraged to behave in skillful and healthy ways toward themselves and others to ensure that rebirth will be as auspicious as possible. Within this view, the spiritual aspect of self consists of de-conditioning mental habits, which lead to the understanding of the interdependent nature of all life, the importance of valuing all life—human and animal, and the intention to treat all sentient beings with utmost compassion and lovingkindness.

Quick and Condensed Definitions of Terms

Anatta—Nonself, the lack of essential or inherent existence of composite things, including the personality.

Anicca—Impermanence of all phenomena.

Buddha—"Awakened mind"; the enduring state of clarity into the nature of reality attained by the Buddha and for which all human beings are encouraged to strive.

Dukkha—The suffering, distress, agony, and so forth that characterizes human existence.

Eightfold Path—Practical advice, contained within the Buddhist sacred texts (e.g., the Dhammapada), describing the importance of maximizing physical and psychological health through skillful perception, thinking, compassion, behavior, speech, livelihood, emotion, meditation, and concentration.

Five Skandhas—The core elements of the self: the physical body, consciousness, cognition–perception, emotion, and conditioned habits, which in interactive interdependence produce the sense of self.

Four Noble Truths—The first major teaching of the Buddha on the nature, cause, and solution to suffering.

Meditation—Training the mind to perceive whatever occurs without exaggeration or distortion.

Nirvana—The state of enlightenment described as the elimination of the conditioned ways of perceiving, thinking, and behaving that lead to suffering.

Prayer

The theistic forms of Buddhism do encourage practitioners to pray for special blessings such as healing of illness, either one's own or that of others. Such prayers may be directed at Buddhist divinities or take the form of meditative contemplations in which Buddhist practitioners themselves are the means by which illness can be healed. Buddhist clergy may also be asked to conduct specific prayer rituals designed to benefit someone who is ill.

However, all Buddhist traditions stress meditation as the key method of self-transformation and personal healing. Prayer may accompany meditation and contemplation primarily as a supportive practice that can enhance meditation. In general, Buddhist prayer is used primarily to awaken one's own compassion and wisdom rather than to petition external forces to bestow blessings.

Religious Calendar

Different Buddhist traditions will celebrate saints and teachers especially significant for that tradition. However, there are several days that are considered sacred across most Buddhist traditions. New Year is celebrated at different times of the year in different traditions, but for most Buddhists, this occurs either on the first full moon in April or the first full moon in January. Vesak, which takes place on the first full moon in May, celebrates the Buddha's birth, death, and attainment of nirvana. These holidays are celebrated through ritual celebrations and readings from the Buddhist teachings in temples and monasteries as well as privately in homes. These celebrations typically include the sharing of a communal meal.

Health-Promoting Practices

Moderation might be considered the key word when describing Buddhist approaches to lifestyle and health promotion. Many, but not all, Buddhists practice vegetarianism. For those who eat meat, as is true for eating any food, one is advised to be moderate. If meat is to be eaten, the Buddhist must neither slaughter the animal nor request that an animal be slaughtered on his or her behalf. Buddhists pay attention to choosing health practices that minimize harm to others or the environment. This may result in favoring locally grown food, minimal use of pesticides or herbicides, and sustainable agriculture. The use of intoxicants is generally proscribed; they may, however, be consumed in moderation, where it is legal to do so. In general, dietary habits reflect the cultural milieu of the Buddhist, rather than unique Buddhist advice.

Healing Rituals

Theistic forms of Buddhism may suggest specific prayers to deities of healing (such as the Medicine Buddha), mantras (special phrases believed to possess special efficacy), visualizations, and meditations. These may be conducted by a Buddhist chaplain or monk, by individuals themselves if they are able, or anyone else who has the required knowledge and devotion. Some forms of Buddhism, such as Tibetan Buddhism, have developed indigenous forms of medical practice, which may be integrated into a Western medical approach. An emphasis may be placed on maintaining a calm and tranquil mind, avoiding extreme states of distress. This approach recognizes that illness may result from a causal process that is ameliorated by increased self-understanding and wisdom. In addition, how one copes with an illness or any adversity can be a means of teaching others about impermanence, suffering, and the lack of essential self—key components of Buddhist wisdom.

Other Unique Religious Beliefs, Rites, and Practices Related to Health or Illness

Tibetan Buddhism has a well-established practice that takes into account the period of time between rebirths. A skilled Buddhist meditation master can guide an individual to the most auspicious rebirth through a series of prayers and meditation.

A belief common across Buddhist traditions is that the onset of illness is an indication of the fruition and culmination of previous causes and actions (possibly originating in previous lives) and thus an excellent opportunity to gain merit through ethical and moral practices in this life. Consequently, one's attitude toward the illness is important and should avoid blaming, self-pity, hopelessness, or victimization. Rather, one is encouraged to utilize the illness as a powerful indicant of Buddhist teachings because illness reminds one of the ultimate impermanence and composite nature of all life.

Unique Religious Beliefs, Rites, and Practices Related to Birthing

There are no specific Buddhist birthing practices. Practices will reflect the various cultural milieus in which Buddhists live.

Unique Religious Beliefs, Rites, or Practices Related to Childrearing

Childrearing practices will generally reflect cultural and personal practices rather than specific Buddhist principles.

Unique Beliefs, Practices, and Rituals Surrounding Dying, Death, and Bereavement

Although beliefs and practices surrounding death may vary across Buddhist traditions, Buddhists will all agree that death is a natural and inevitable event that points to the inherent impermanence of everything—including the human body. The dying process is encouraged to be as calm, meditative, and reflective as possible. This is both a means to facilitate an auspicious rebirth and to teaching others who are present about central Buddhist beliefs about impermanence. If possible, the dying individual may meditate on specific forms of the Buddha (such as the Medicine Buddha or the Buddha of Compassion, Avalokitsheshvara) or engage in specific liturgical practices during the dying process. Following physical death, most traditions will engage in ritual prayer and meditation to ensure that the deceased individual will obtain a favorable rebirth.

Thus, the end of this life heralds the beginning of another life that, while it cannot be taken as the direct continuation of the personality that was just deceased, will bear the strong influence of the previous birth. While the specific rebirth will depend to a large extent on the deceased person's character and behavior, the spiritual community can assist—through prayer, meditation, and ritual—to ensure that the optimal rebirth takes place by mitigating any obstacles to an auspicious rebirth.

Role of Religious Community (Persons or Organizations) During Health Challenges

All Buddhist traditions hold regular, at least weekly, formal events at temples or monasteries. At these events, attendees may practice meditation, recite prayers and liturgies, chant mantras and devotional songs, receive teachings from the Buddhist canon, celebrate special holidays, consult with clergy, share a communal meal, and so forth. Depending on the tradition, these rituals may involve special devotional practices dedicated to specific Buddhist deities, whereas others may primarily emphasize intensive meditation and contemplation. Because many of these religious practices can take place anywhere, an individual who is unable to go to a temple or monastery can do them privately.

Role of Clergy During Health Challenges

Buddhist clergy will make hospital and home visits to comfort the sick individual. Clergy will provide reassurance, compassion, prayer, instruction, and other aspects of Buddhist spiritual practice to congregation members facing illness and death.

Unique Religious Aspects of Family Involvement

Illness can be viewed as a time for family members to resolve conflicts, express compassion, and derive wisdom on the nature of human life. (After all, the Buddha said that life is characterized ultimately by aging, illness, and death.) Thus, illness is viewed as a natural life process that can teach those who are witnessing a family member's illness important insights about their own nature. In addition, family members can all participate in any of the religious aspects associated with healing, such as prayer, mantra, visualization, meditation, and liturgy. Often, family members are encouraged to engage in these activities on their own time and whenever they can devote time to healing rituals.

Nursing Implications Unique to This Religious Tradition

- Buddhist spiritual practices strengthen the believer's positive attitude and equanimity amidst the threat of illness or death. Ensure Buddhist patients have periods of uninterrupted calm for meditation and other healing practices, as well as clergy visits.

- Ways nurses can support Buddhist patients to meditate also include offering to bring recorded meditations and chants, liturgical texts, meditation cushion, Buddhist images and iconography, rosaries or yantras, and providing a quiet time and space to allow the patient to practice in a way that is meaningful to them.

- The dying process is encouraged to be as calm and reflective as possible so as to facilitate an auspicious rebirth. It is particularly important to Buddhists to have Buddhist clergy support around the time of death who can offer chants and meditations to foster calmness and a positive rebirth. If a Buddhist patient is actively dying, confirm with the family or your institution's spiritual care service that a Buddhist chaplain or clergy has been notified. The Buddhist Chaplains Network is an on-line community of Buddhist chaplains committed to spiritual care giving (www. buddhistchaplainsnetwork.org). A directory of Buddhist chaplains throughout the United States can be found at www.buddhistchaplains.org.

- While many Buddhists are vegetarian, the more important and prevalent dietary practice is that of having moderation in all things.

- Given the different streams of Buddhism, it is important to assess what health care–related beliefs and practices are important to each Buddhist patient. Some may not go to temples, have clergy, pray, or observe many religious rituals. Not all Buddhists, of course, are ascetics.

- Remember that even though a Buddhist patient might meditate and remain calm in the midst of suffering, this does not mean they are not suffering and feeling the pain of impermanence.

FOR MORE INFORMATION

Visit www.accesstoinsight.org for a comprehensive listing of all of the Buddha's teachings with commentaries by prominent Buddhist scholars.
Visit www.buddhanet.com for information about all Buddhist traditions.
Chodron, T. (2001). *Buddhism for beginners*. Ithaca, NY: Snow Lion Publications.
Hanh, T. N. (1999). *The heart of the Buddha's teaching*. New York, NY: Three Rivers Press.

13 Christian Scientists

CONTRIBUTOR: *Linda Kohler*
REVIEWER: *Russ Gerber*

Theology and Social History

Mary Baker Eddy wrote that she found Christian Science (CS) in the Bible. She was born into a deeply religious Christian household in New England in 1821. In her mid-40s, she was so severely injured in a fall that she was not expected to recover. Using her Bible, she experienced a profound moment of spiritual insight and was immediately restored to health. She spent the next several years immersed in studying the Bible to discover the method of healing that she felt had healed her that day. During this time, she wrote a book called *Science and Health With Key to the Scriptures*, which explained the method or principles of prayer-based Christian healing, which she called CS. In the 140 years since, CS has spread primarily through healing.

People came to Mary Baker Eddy first seeking healing and then to learn from her how to heal others through applying the same Bible-based principles. As her students took this teaching to their communities, churches were formed as a place to share the teachings and to encourage one another in the healing application of CS. By the time Mary Baker Eddy passed away (1910), she left a well-established church structure that provides for the ongoing spiritual education and daily devotional study of anyone wishing to investigate or use CS. CS congregations tend to focus their energies on the daily application of CS in their lives and on praying for individual, community, and world issues that need healing. Each local church maintains a CS Reading Room as an outreach to the community and a resource to members for their own self-study. The Church also publishes *The Christian Science Monitor*, which many members see as an agenda for their prayers for the world.

The early church, centered in Boston, Massachusetts, spread rapidly throughout the United States and Canada in the late 1800s as well as in Europe (especially England and Germany) in the early 1900s. The religion initially grew mostly in English-speaking areas given study of the textbook, *Science and Health*, which is essential to its practice. Translations of *Science and Health* are now published in 16 additional languages. Today, church members reside in 130 countries, and 72 countries have "branch" churches or societies, with the largest concentration of members and branches in the United States.

Christian Science is a Christian religion, based upon the Old and New Testaments of the Christian Bible. Christian Science is not, nor is it related to, Scientology or faith healing. CS theology speaks to a spiritual approach to life rather than to any particular social, economic, or educational orientation. The Church does not advise, formally or informally, its members regarding health care decisions.

Deity/God or Ultimate Other

CS is monotheistic and emphasizes the First Commandment of Moses— one God—and defines God as "The great I AM; the all-knowing, all-seeing, all-acting, all-wise, all-loving, and eternal; Principle; Mind; Soul; Spirit; Life; Truth; Love; all substance; intelligence" (*Science and Health*, p. 587). CS also refers to God as "Father–Mother" and teaches that God, as a loving Father, provides for, guides, and protects His children. As Mother, God tenderly cares for, nurtures, cherishes, and nourishes Her children. God is love and wants only good for each of us. Humanity's relative ignorance of God, rather than any unwillingness or incapacity on God's part, would tend to make one feel cut off from this constant, loving care.

Views on Health and Well-Being

Health is understood to be more than freedom from physical symptoms. A healthy body is a natural by-product of spiritual mindedness (compassion, truthfulness, forgiveness, fearlessness, and so forth). Consistently loving God and loving one's neighbor improves one's mental state. This spiritual mindedness, in turn, improves one's overall health.

Explanations for Disease and Illness

Many studies today acknowledge a link between thought and health—a "mind/body" connection. Most people are aware of placebo and nocicebo effects, as well, showing the relation of beliefs and expectations to outcomes. Experience has shown that as spiritual mindedness brings hope and freedom and thus produces a positive effect on the body. Conversely, fear, uncertainty, and anger can be harmful to health of both mind and body.

The Nature of Suffering and How to Address It

Suffering is not viewed as a punishment from God or as an inevitable human condition. Suffering is to be alleviated and healed. The spiritual truths rooted in the Bible and promoted in CS have a liberating and strengthening effect on human lives. Relief from physical or emotional suffering comes quickly when one turns to God in prayer.

Death, Dying, and Afterlife

Death is an enemy (see 1 Corinthians 15:26). Death is not something to accept or to prepare for but to triumph over. Not that when a Christian Scientist dies this indicates they have failed to live up to the teachings of the religion, but simply that the ideal is to triumph over "the last enemy." A Christian Scientist is comforted by reminders of God sending "angels" to keep persons safe (e.g., Psalm 91). Angels are viewed as thoughts that come from God that inspire and strengthen persons. These "angels" bring comfort and healing.

Quick and Condensed Definitions of Terms

CS practitioner—an experienced Christian Scientist whose full-time vocation is providing CS treatment to others. They will generally make hospital or house calls if asked.

CS treatment—a specific form of mental and spiritual treatment that eradicates the fear of or submission to suffering which, in turn, is detrimental to health. This treatment is based on the love, power, and presence of an all-good God. The practitioner does not have to be present with the patient to give such treatment, which can last a moment or many hours.

Prayer

Prayer is central to the Christian Scientist's quest for healing. It is a common, almost constant practice. An important aspect of communication with God involves cultivating one's own innate receptivity to God as Spirit. We are meant to listen, understand, and accept God's care. Jesus taught the qualities of thought that tend toward this receptivity: humility, gratitude, forgiveness, compassion, faith. Study of the Bible and *Science and Health*, prayer, worship, and living consistently with one's prayers open the heart to a clearer understanding and acceptance of what God is communicating.

Christian Scientists (CSs) generally begin each day with devotional reading of the Bible and *Science and Health*, studying a regular Bible lesson, as well as applying what they learn to themselves, their families, and the world. Christian Scientists make a distinction between this type of general prayer and CS treatment, which is provided upon individual request. While Christian Scientists may pray in a general way for everyone, CS treatment is specific help, usually for an individual, and relates to a specific problem or need.

Religious Calendar

Sunday morning worship services and midweek testimony meetings are important opportunities to receive spiritual refreshment and to give gratitude for blessings received. The only additional special religious service is held on Thanksgiving Day. Gratitude is extremely important to Christian Scientists. They know it to be a powerful impetus for healing.

Health-Promoting Practices

The CS Church does not prohibit or require any specific lifestyle practices. *Science and Health* teaches that daily prayer for oneself and obedience to the moral teachings of the Bible are healthy and wise choices. Members are highly individual in how they apply this teaching.

Healing Rituals

CS is largely free of outward religious rituals. For example, baptism and communion are seen as deeply personal spiritual experiences—purification of thought and spiritual communion with God. Rather, inspiration and healing can come from the Daily Bible Lesson (available in print, audio, and digital products) and additional study and prayer at intervals throughout the day. Sources that encourage this study and prayer include:

- the Bible or *Science and Health* (audio books are available at a CS Reading Room or ask a family member to locate them for you);

- other writings by Mary Baker Eddy;

- CS periodicals—*The Christian Science Journal* (monthly) and *Christian Science Sentinel* (weekly); many articles are reprinted online at spirituality.com, and themed audio collections of articles are available on CD at CS Reading Rooms;

- a CS practitioner (try to arrange for privacy for this visit);

- Sunday Church Services and midweek testimony meetings (available live or as a rebroadcast at christianscience.com); and

- hymns (patients will appreciate hymns that are specific to CS, as distinctions in semantics can be important; CDs are available at CS Reading Rooms).

Other Unique Religious Beliefs, Rites, and Practices Related to Health or Illness

Christian Scientists tend not to want to hear a lot about their symptoms, diagnosis, or prognosis. They are trying to look away from the disease model and keep thought focused on the spiritual ideas about which they are praying. Most Christian Scientists will either decline or be highly selective in their acceptance of medical examinations, procedures, medications, therapies, diets, and so forth. This is not in response to an imposed dogma. Rather, it is because CS treatment and medical treatment have differing expectations; medical methods could interfere with or undermine the desired outcomes of a Christian Scientist. Christian Scientists are free to make their own decisions about health care needs and typically favor CS treatment because it has proven itself effective throughout their lives.

Consequently, Christian Scientists may ask for discharge, which allopathic practitioners consider premature. If they will need skilled care, it may be possible to locate a CS nursing facility or private CS nurse who could care for them in their home. Such nurses provide skillful physical care without medications or medical procedures and, because they are themselves Christian Scientists, bring a unique degree of sensitivity to the patient's health care.

Unique Religious Beliefs, Rites, and Practices Related to Birthing

Christian Scientist parents may be selective about accepting tests, procedures, or treatments that allopathic clinicians may consider routine. Birthing mothers may decline anesthesia. (Many CS mothers have experienced painless or relatively pain-free childbirth and attribute this to prayer.) The parents may want a CS practitioner or nurse to be present at the birth. Neither would be there to assist with the mechanical aspects of the birth. A CS practitioner would be present if immediate need for CS treatment occurred. A CS nurse would be present to support the mother during the birth and to care for the mother and child once the doctor or midwife completed their work.

Circumcision is an individual choice. Some will decline, some will not.

Unique Religious Beliefs, Rites, or Practices Related to Childrearing

Christian Scientist parents may request exemption from physical examination and immunization for their children. This is not a passive choice. These parents pray daily for the safety and well-being of their children. Whereas these parents would turn to medical care for a child if needed, they generally find CS treatment to be highly effective in caring for their child's health and well-being.

Unique Beliefs, Practices, and Rituals Surrounding Dying, Death, and Bereavement

Christian Scientists will generally prefer the least invasive and most respectful option for postmortem care or examination.

Role of Religious Community (Persons or Organizations) During Health Challenges

Christian Scientists meet weekly in community in church auditoriums, Reading Rooms, or public meeting spaces. Sunday church services include readings from the Bible, hymns, prayers, and fellowship. Wednesday midweek testimony meetings allow the congregation to meet for an hour to hear readings and to give thanks for the blessings and healing experiences. Services and midweek meetings at The Mother Church in Boston (worldwide headquarters of the CS church) are broadcast live over the Internet, so it is possible for anyone with an internet connection (or even an iPhone) to listen to them live or rebroadcast (found at christianscience.com.). Although church services generally include a time for collective silent prayer, Christian Scientists tend to not ask the church as a group to pray for them in times of illness. Instead, they prefer to seek help confidentially through the practice of an experienced Christian Scientist.

Although there is no formal social services network within the church, nursing support for Christian Scientists is available. Individual CS nurses are located through *The Christian Science Journal* Directory (online at christianscience.force.com/AdvDirectoryLookup). Some areas have a "Visiting Christian Science Nursing Service" and/or a CS Nursing Facility (online directory of facilities available at aocsn.org). Support is often arranged through a local branch of Church of Christ, Scientist; some branches have committees to organize these visits, whereas others will simply respond spontaneously to a need. You can do a geographical search of churches online at christianscience.force.com/AdvDirectoryLookup.

Role of Clergy During Health Challenges

Laypersons (e.g., "readers") lead congregations rather than credentialed clergy. Church members who may support patients include CS nurses and practitioners.

Unique Religious Aspects of Family Involvement

Some Christian Scientists (not all) are extremely private about their health issues. They may not want visits (or may want to keep them short) from friends and even family members who are not Christian Scientists. They may choose to notify some and not other family members, probably preferring ones who will understand and support whatever care choices they have made. In any dire health circumstance, family emotions can become intense. If family members disagree about what treatment options to choose because of religious interpretations, it is vital to remember that all do ultimately want what is best for the loved one who is in extremis.

Nursing Implications Unique to This Religious Tradition

- CS practitioners and nurses can be contacted via phone or email. Consult christianscience.force.com/AdvDirectoryLookup or a phone directory to find a local church or Reading Room where you can obtain information about local practitioners and nurses.

- Christian Scientists normally exercise a high degree of individual responsibility in caring for themselves. Sometimes this individualism comes out as a bit of a stubborn streak in older members who are struggling to preserve their independence and privacy.

- Refusal of medical care is not because of adherence to any church rulings. Rather, it is free choice of preference for a paradigm that respects that spiritual healing effects physical and mental healing.

FOR MORE INFORMATION

Visit www.christianscience.com or visit a Christian Science Reading Room.
Eddy, M. B. (2000). *Science and health with key to the Scriptures.* Boston, MA: Christian Science Board of Directors.

14 Hindus

CONTRIBUTOR: *Shukavak Dasa, PhD*
NURSE REVIEWER: *Rani Srivastava, PhD, RN*

Theology and Social History

The world's third largest faith tradition is possibly the oldest in existence, with sacred texts dating back to as early as 1700 BCE. Although Hindus primarily live in the Indian subcontinent, the diaspora has spread considerably to North America and the United Kingdom. Hinduism is an ethnic religion, not a religion with an organized ecclesiastical structure based on creeds.

Although there are various denominations within Hinduism, there are some fundamentals that most Hindu adherents would accept. These include the authority of the *Vedas* (oldest sacred texts); the law of karma, which determines one's destiny in this and future lives; transmigration of souls from one body to another (i.e., after death, the soul is reincarnated); and the ultimate goal desired is release from the cycle of death and rebirth (*moksha*). Although most Hindus believe in one ultimate being or God, there is wide variation in beliefs among Hindus regarding how their God/s are manifested.

For the Hindu, there are four primary purposes or objectives in life. These include *dharma* (living righteously and practicing spiritual disciplines that lead one to God), *artha* (having a livelihood and prospering), and *kama* (enjoying sensual pleasures). Ultimately, the goal for all is *moksha* (enlightenment) that variously means union with God, being in the presence of God, the self-realization of God within, mental peace, or realizing the unity of all existence. During one's lifespan as these primary goals are pursued, one passes through four stages (*ashramas*): (1) study, learning spiritual knowledge; (2) generative work (e.g., marrying, procreating, professional endeavoring, supporting family and others); (3) retirement, during which one gives back to one's community and gradually detaches from the material world (e.g., volunteers, begins to give possessions away); and (4) asceticism, when in old age one readies for *moksha* by giving up all desires and becoming totally devoted to God.

These religious values and principles guiding the Hindu way of life emanate from many sacred writings. The original sacred texts are the *Vedas*. Guiding everyday life are the *Bhagavad Gita* (or *Gita*) and *Ramayana*. These texts include epic narratives and prose.

Deity/God or Ultimate Other

Devout Hindus seek an awareness of God in daily life. For some, God is personal, whereas for others, God is an infinite principle. Although Hindus believe in one Supreme Being, *Brahman*, there are thousands of representations of this Ultimate Reality. Because *Brahman* is infinite, intangible, genderless, eternal, and beyond human understanding, *Brahman* can be represented by a multiplicity of Gods and Goddesses, each of which is linked with certain qualities (e.g., wealth, fertility, art, wisdom). Incarnated forms of God who have appeared at different times in human history include *Rama* and *Krishna*. These many deities worshipped are all manifestations of one omnipotent, omniscient, and omnipresent God. Thus, Hindus are both polytheistic and monotheistic concurrently. Although Hindus are free to worship any deities, the prevalence and preferences for worshipping certain deities fall along denominational lines.

Views on Health and Well-Being

Health involves the balance of mind, body, and soul with nature. Although Hinduism views health holistically, the relationships among the components are understood differently than in Western theories. The biggest difference is that consciousness is associated with the soul, not the mind.

Health is also determined by the law of *karma*. That is, the actions and deeds lead to good or bad reactions—in this life or the next. Health is also both personal and social and requires actions aimed at preserving personal as well as social morality.

A Hindu scientific approach to a healthy life is found in *Ayurvedic* medicine. This extensive body of knowledge, which offers information about how to promote health and prevent and cure disease, is recognized internationally. *Ayurveda's* scientific approach reflects Hindu philosophy, which posits the universe is made of five basic elements: earth (*prithvi*), water (*jala*), fire (*teja*), air (*vayu*), and ether or space (*akash*). Of these elements, the three that interact in the human body to determine health are body of wind, fire, and water (existing in the forms of breath, bile, and mucus). The balance of these three body elements, although affected by seasons, climate, hygiene, and one's constitution, determines health.

Because balance is vital to health, importance is given to moderation in eating, sleeping, having sexual intercourse, and taking medicine. *Ayurvedic* theory also emphasizes the functions of metabolism, digestion, and excretion in maintaining health. *Ayurvedic* medicinal treatments include exercise, yoga, meditation, massage, steaming, and herbs.

Explanations for Disease and Illness

Illness is viewed holistically; physical and mental illness are seen as strongly connected. Hindus attach considerable importance to the relationship between the mind (mental activities) and the body (physical functions). Any disturbance in one affects the other and causes diseases. Mental activities such as grief, fear, worry, anger, and sorrow are recognized as causative factors for physical illness, such as indigestion. Therefore, for maintaining one's health as well as for curing disease, it is required that both the mind and the body are kept in proper condition.

As explained above, an imbalance in the body elements also contributes to disease. To restore balance, a holistic treatment includes medicine, diet, keeping proper daily routines, spiritual and scriptural knowledge, patience, prayer, and meditation. Wrongful actions also create stress intrapersonally and interpersonally, contributing to personal and social illness.

The destiny that results from *karma* also explains disease and illness. Given the law of karma, although what happens to someone in the present is to some extent unchangeable and beyond control, one's chosen response will influence what occurs in the future. Hindus may also ascribe curses or the "evil eye" as causes of disease. "Evil eye," or *nazzar,* can be cast intentionally or unintentionally when one is subject to great admiration.

The Nature of Suffering and How to Address It

A Hindu patient may view illness as karma and rely on the principles of *dharma* to respond to it. For those accepting that everything that happens is a result of karma, illness is not random. Thus, questions like "why me?" can easily be answered with "it is karma." Suffering can be seen as a way of voiding the effects of past negative *karma*; it is also an opportunity to be tested and learn from the difficult experience. Acceptance of suffering can indicate progress toward *moksha*. For example, although attributions are multifaceted, if a patient is diagnosed with a chronic or serious illness, it may be considered that it is because of past deeds that caused suffering to others; it may also be so the patient can develop spiritual qualities. (When children become seriously ill, the sickness is often attributed to past parental or ancestral actions. Thus, parents of seriously ill children suffer because of this as well as worry about its effect on lineage.) Comfort is also found in remembering that even if the body is hurt, the soul is not harmed. A Hindu will try to respond to suffering by controlling mental stress (e.g., fear, anxiety) because it would aggravate disease.

Death, Dying, and Afterlife

In Hinduism, the soul is the central entity. It is not the body that has a soul, but rather, the soul has a body. So when the soul leaves, the body ceases to function, and death occurs. Death, however, is not forever as the eternal soul is part of *Brahman,* the Absolute Being. Hindus believe that existence is eternal and that each life is a cycle in the ongoing journey or quest toward *moksha*. *Moksha* is the release from the human condition and *karma* (good or bad) and into a condition where time and space cease to exist and all is seen as one.

Quick and Condensed Definitions of Terms

Atmaan—Individual self or the eternal soul, which is identical to Brahman in essence.

Ayurveda—A traditional system of medicine, regarded as the Hindu science of healing.

Bhagavad Gita—Literally translated as the song of God, the *Gita* is sacred Hindu text considered to be a concise guide to Hindu theology and a practical guide to life.

Brahman—Absolute God.

Dharma—Divine law or path of righteousness that involves (in part) detachment from material things and relationships so as to ultimately find unity with *Brahman*.

Ishwar—Another name for God.

Karma—Literally means "actions or deeds." In Hinduism, karma refers to the law of causality where actions or deeds (whether voluntary or involuntary) lead to beneficial or harmful effects. The effects may not be immediate but are accumulative and may be experienced later in one's current life or in subsequent lives. The end result of karma is that a soul gains a variety of experiences and wisdom over a series of lives and eventually sees the world as God does. Karma can also be good and positive, and rewards in this life are considered the result of gains made in the last. Karma is everything that one has ever thought, spoken, done, or caused (intentionally or unintentionally) and is also that which one thinks, speaks, or does this very moment. Thus, karma is not imposed by outside forces, either by God or by a punitive force, and it is not fate, as humans act with free will and therefore create their own destiny. Instead, it is accumulated through one's thoughts, words, and actions and throughout the various cycles of birth and re-birth.

Moksha—Release from cycle of birth and death. In *moksha*, there is ultimate peace, ultimate knowledge, and ultimate enlightenment.

Prayer

Prayer is the recitation of mantras. These mantras (especially those for circumstances such as illness) are passages from holy scriptures prescribed by the priest who selects the mantra after consulting a horoscope. Astrology will also guide the priest to prescribe what type of vow the person may make to petition a god. For example, one may vow to perform a religious ritual (*puja*), so many times during a time period, or wear a ring with a gem representing the planet aligned with the astrological recommendation, or one may vow to fast (generally done only by women who desire health for a family member) or not to eat certain foods (e.g., salt). Hindus personify their gods. This means that if the god can be befriended and flattered with vows, one is most likely to receive the requested favor.

Hindus may also practice meditation or yoga to develop spiritual discipline. Meditation may involve a soft or silent chanting of a mantra while in the "Lotus position," whereas yoga involves meditation while breathing deeply and exercising a special posture.

Devout Hindus will recite mantras, sing, chant, and/or meditate each morning. They may have a family shrine in the home, which has a tangible image (icon) of god/s. Worship may also include lighting a candle and offering fruit or flowers to their deity.

Religious Calendar

Many holy days or festivals occur each year (which follows a lunar calendar). These festivals celebrate events from Hindu mythology and are often observed with social events.

There are days or times that are considered to be either auspicious or inauspicious for critical events (e.g., marriages). Performing religious rituals and significant health-related procedures (e.g., surgery, discontinuing life support) at auspicious times is important.

Health-Promoting Practices

Hindus believe that it is important to keep mind, body, and environment pure and free of wrongdoing or toxins. Purity of body is maintained through strict hygienic practices. Purity of mind creates trust and results from good intentions. One way Hindus strive for purity is by regular bathing. Saliva and body discharges are considered to be impure and polluting (*tamsic*); in addition, menstruation is seen as very polluting. When one is in an impure state, there may be a need for restrictions from particular activities or additional rituals to counter the impurity.

Many traditional Hindus will first treat symptoms with home remedies such as massage, bathing, and herbal medicines. These and other Ayurvedic therapies are used to promote health and heal illness.

Healing Rituals

A family member may ask a priest for a *puja* at the temple. The priest will say a mantra that incorporates the patient's name. Incense, candles, or oil lamps are waved, and fruit or flowers offered before the image of the deity. The priest will then give the family member temple food, a remnant of sacred cloth (e.g., to be placed on the bed or worn around the shoulders), or something tangible to return to the prayed-for patient.

Often, rituals symbolizing purification are practiced after some life events (e.g., birthing, mourning, hospitalization). These rituals typically involve a symbolic cleansing with water, purification by fire, and chanting prayers or mantras. The rituals may be facilitated by a priest or a family elder.

Other Unique Religious Beliefs, Rites, and Practices Related to Health or Illness

Although tea is a staple, Hindus generally do not consume caffeinated or alcoholic drinks.

Sometimes, Hindus may be hesitant to use medicines as they may perceive taking them is inconsistent with acceptance and suffering.

Unique Religious Beliefs, Rites, and Practices Related to Birthing

Procreation is considered a duty and the reason for marriage and sexual intercourse. There are particular ceremonies and foods, as well as limitations in activities, for the mother during the childbearing stage. There are also a number of rituals that are performed when the baby is born for the purity and welfare of the mother and child.

Because all life is sacred and must be allowed to fulfill its destiny, abortion is never an option.

Circumcision is never done.

Unique Religious Beliefs, Rites, or Practices Related to Childrearing

Special ceremonies occur at significant times in a child's life. When a baby is born, it is welcomed into the world with ghee and honey placed on the tongue, an ear pierced, and the father whispering the name of God into the infant's ear. Other ceremonies exist when the child is named, first fed solid food around 6 months of age, and for those in the three upper castes, at the first haircut. Between the ages of 7 and 11, boys celebrate a "thread ceremony," a rite of passage signifying entry to adulthood when they receive a blessed thread that they will always wear.

Traditionally, it is the role of the family (especially the elders) to ensure children receive religious instruction. Children may receive instruction from a guru (teacher), an expert on spiritual knowledge.

Unique Beliefs, Practices, and Rituals Surrounding Dying, Death, and Bereavement

Hindus will prefer to die at home and under circumstances where they have control. Death is not to be hurried or resisted as an enemy of life as it is requisite to rebirthing and journeying toward the ultimate destination of *moksha*. However, this does not mean a Hindu would always refuse resuscitation or life support. Unless a patient is actively dying, extraordinary means are not prohibited. It is also inappropriate to predict when death will occur, as the suggestive power in doing so may invite death prematurely.

When death is imminent, a priest will be called to perform a religious ritual. After the death, the family will likely want to participate in washing the body of the deceased. Holy ash or some organic paste will be applied to the deceased's forehead, and a few drops of holy water will be instilled in the mouth. Some may want to place the body facing south (toward the god of death). Hindus prefer cremation within 24 hours of death and generally do not embalm the dead.

A number of days of mourning (10–40) ensue. Grief is absorbed by the family of the deceased. That is, because of the association with death, the family is considered to be in a polluted state. There may be restrictions on when food can be cooked at home and other rituals, which can be performed at home or at a temple for the peaceful transition of the soul and the family's comfort.

Role of Religious Community (Persons or Organizations) During Health Challenges

Hindus are not obligated to visit a temple. They may visit the temple for a meeting and do a *puja* with others on holy festival days or regularly (e.g., every Sunday in North America). Although the particular day of the week varies with the diety worshiped, Tuesday is a more sacred day than others for most Hindus. The temple *puja* can include singing mantras or partaking of a sacred meal. A family may have a *puja* at home or at the temple for special occasions. The activities of temples in Western countries often reflect the Western holidays as well (e.g., have a *puja* on New Year's Day, January 1).

Like the patient or family, the Hindu community may pray, fast, and perform other rituals on behalf of the sick. Temples do not have persons or organized groups to care for the sick. However, as the Hindu population in the West increases, they are increasingly developing social services of their own (e.g., Society for Battered Women). These nascent services are limited to a local area.

Role of Clergy During Health Challenges

Although priests are not expected to visit the sick, a patient's family member may seek out a priest at the local temple. Generally, the only time a priest would be summoned to perform a ritual is at the time of death. A priest functions as a shaman. A priest (or several, if petition for god is serious) may also be hired by a family to recite mantras for their sick member.

Unique Religious Aspects of Family Involvement

The nuclear and extended family of Hindu patients will pay extended visits to their sick and are quite involved in direct care. If permitted, they often bring their loved one food. It is typical for the family to be involved in washing the body after a loved one has died. The obligation to give care to a parent generally falls to the sons (and hence, daughters-in-law). Modern societies, however, are changing these traditions; families are increasingly becoming reliant on nonfamily members' help.

Nursing Implications Unique to This Religious Tradition

• The degree to which Hindus accept traditional beliefs and practices will vary with how assimilated and educated in Western culture they are. Thus, variations in beliefs (e.g., about the cause of disease and how to treat it) can exist within a family—between and within generations.

• The importance of purity is manifested symbolically and literally in various ways in the life of a Hindu. For example, often Hindus will take off their shoes when entering a home—or hospital room. They do not hand things to another using the left hand (historically associated with use for unclean body areas). Before a meal, water is sprinkled around the plate in an act of purification. This desire for purity also translates into daily practice in the habit of regular bathing, especially in the morning. Meals are eaten after the mouth and teeth are cleaned (unlike in Western hospitals, where breakfast is offered first and morning care later).

• How and what a Hindu eats may reflect traditional practices. That is, food is eaten only after it has been offered first to god/s. In addition to sprinkling water around the plate, five morsels may be left on the table to recognize one's indebtedness to the divine. The foods eaten are, ideally, those which create inner purity, clear mind, calmness, and health. Thus, foods that may be avoided include garlic and onion, salt and strong spices, eggs and commercially made cheese, as well as old or overripe food. Meat (especially beef and possibly pork) is never eaten. Because of respect for the sacred life of these animals, many Hindus are vegetarians. Even nonvegetarians may observe a vegetarian diet on particular days of the week, festivals, or times of the year. Fruits, vegetables, grains, and nuts are considered to be the most healthful of foods. Moderation in the amount of food consumed is recommended.

• A sacred thread may be worn around the neck or chest under clothing. When sick, a thread blessed by a priest may be placed around the wrist or upper arm, or a protective verse from scripture kept in a silver container on a chain may be worn. These talismans should not be cut or removed unless agreed upon with the patient or family, as they are to ward off the evil force possibly causing the disease. Likewise, a woman's marriage, symbolized by gold jewelry or a red dot worn on the forehead, should not be removed unless permission is obtained.

- Hindus view freedom of religion as the freedom to not be proselytized. However, they may appreciate the opportunity to talk about God, given the belief that there is ultimately one God, albeit different paths to God.

- Modesty is very important to Hindus. For intimate procedures (e.g., enemas), ask the patient if a nurse of the same gender is preferred. If this is not possible, ask the patient if they would like the spouse or a family member to be present. Offer older women as long a gown as possible.

- Traditional Hindu elders are likely to take a passive role in health care decision making. This may manifest in not asking any questions, yet being very cooperative in providing information. The decision making may be assumed by the family, especially its male members. Decisions may also be influenced by the extent to which a patient will still be able to carry out desired practices and rituals that are seen as being a critical part of one's *dharmic* life.

- When a Hindu is initially prescribed a medication, assess for herbal and homeopathic treatments that may be contraindicated with the new medication. Also, evaluate the patient's attitude toward taking the medicine, as some may perceive Western health care overmedicates patients.

- Whereas receiving guidance from elders and others who are wise is basic to Hindus, Western counseling for mental illness may be resisted if it views the illness as purely a mind problem and does not offer a holistic approach to treatment.

- Recitation of relevant *Vedic* hymns is important at significant times in one's life, such as birth, marriage, death, or the start of a new venture. This recitation may be done silently or softly while alone or in community with family at home or at the temple.

- Hindus' beliefs about karma can be misinterpreted as fatalism or passivity. However, although the Hindu is to accept circumstances, this does not mean abdicating duty to conduct one's life in the best way possible. Remembering present choices will affect their futures (karmic law) may inspire a patient to rally.

- Whereas the nursing terminology of "spiritual distress" is likely embarrassing for any patient, it does not make sense to a Hindu, as the spirit or soul by nature does not have distress. Instead, it is the mind that may need help.

- Socioculturally, Hindus are collectivists (rather than individualists). The sick will have many visitors, and family will be eager to provide care.

FOR MORE INFORMATION

Visit http://www.religiousportal.com/HinduChildbirth.html (about rituals related to children), and http://www.stanford.edu/group/ethnoger/asianindian.html, http://www.angelfire.com/az/ambersukumaran/medicine.html, http://info .kyha.com/documents/CG-Hindu.pdf (information for health care professionals).

Srivastava, R., Srivastava, B., & Srivastava, R. (2011). Hinduism and nursing. In M. D. Fowler, S. Reimer-Kirkham, R. Sawatzky, & E. J. Taylor (Eds.), *Religion, religious ethics, and nursing* (pp. 173–196). New York, NY: Springer Publishing Company.

15 IFCA International Christians*

CONTRIBUTOR: *The Reverend Joseph Smith*

NURSE REVIEWER: *Patricia Gregory, RN*

Theology and Social History

The Independent Fundamental Churches of America (IFCA) International began with a meeting in Cicero, Illinois, in 1930 where pastors of several Protestant denominations noted that belief in basic Christian views was being challenged by denominational leaders. These basic core values (then called Fundamentals) were more important to them than their denominational distinctives. Because the mainstream Christian church authorities of that time punished those who opposed the intent of the denominational founders, these pastors joined together to give birth to a fellowship—the IFCA. Some others, although just as discouraged by denominational directions, became independent without affiliating with the IFCA. The founders of the IFCA saw a need to project a consistent stance without denominational control. It served as an accrediting association as well as a place for cooperation of like-minded churches.

With the passage of time, this name became inadequate. Institutional freedom had led to more actual interdependence, Fundamental had ceased to mean basic (rather, it had acquired the pejorative meaning of backward), institutional membership was no longer limited to churches, and geographical boundaries were no longer national. All four parts of the name no longer communicated the position of this family of churches. So in recognition of both history and progress, the name was changed in 1996 to IFCA International.

The doctrines did not change, but the same cannot be said of unaffiliated independent churches. With the rise of the "mega-church" (with congregations in the thousands), many of these unaffiliated IFCA churches became so comfortable in their size that they did not see the value of affiliation with IFCA International. Their unwillingness to submit to doctrinal scrutiny produced doctrinal diversity too varied for description here. IFCA International is the only association of independent churches where a common doctrinal position can be found.

Independent Christian churches have existed for centuries. Currently, there are other independent churches with similar characteristics to those of the IFCA International (e.g., some Baptists, the Association of Free

Lutheran Congregations). This chapter will not try to characterize these positions. Local IFCA International churches are typically named "Bible Churches" (e.g., Calvary Bible Church).

Deity/God or Ultimate Other

Those who attend IFCA churches worship the God of the Bible. He is personal, able to reveal Himself, and constantly concerned with the fate of His creation. He primarily communicates to us in the Bible, which was produced as men were moved by the Holy Spirit. We primarily communicate with Him through prayer. He is always ready to hear the prayers of those who believe in Him and is "touched with the feelings of our infirmities."

God leads us individually by His Holy Spirit, as we surrender our wills to Him. Such leading, however, is always to be tried against the Bible. Daily personal direction not spelled out in Scripture is not binding on other individuals. It is designed primarily to foster an intimate relationship between faithful persons and their God as they walk the path He has chosen for them. Patients have full freedom to discern before God the course of treatment they believe will honor God; there are no religious constraints on treatment.

Views on Health and Well-Being

One Biblical concept of wellness we embrace is illustrated in Jesus' question, "Will you be made whole?" Integration of all parts of a person—spirit, soul, mind, and body is the goal of wellness. Another way of thinking about wellness is that it involves restoration from the effects of the fall of mankind, given sin has caused calamity. However, we do not believe that most sickness is the result of personal sin.

The Bible teaches that the body of a believer is a "temple" in which God dwells. Care for the body in both prevention of disease as well as treatment of disease reflects a God-given instinct to honor what belongs to Him.

Explanations for Disease and Illness

Like all earthly evil, illness is a result of the fall of man. It is experienced by both the righteous and the wicked because we live in a fallen world. However, in the case of the righteous, it provides an opportunity to learn patience, compassion, and dependence on a sovereign God. For the wicked, illness produces questions about culpability, accountability, and the meaning of life, sensitizing the soul to deal with the issues of mortality. Illness may result naturally from environmental causes that reflect the general sinfulness of humanity. Illness is caused by personal sin only when it results from unhealthful practices. Not all risky unhealthful behavior, however, causes illness.

The Nature of Suffering and How to Address It

Suffering is allowed to happen to anyone, even those who love God and those who live healthfully. Suffering allows one to experience the comfort of God and share that consolation with others who suffer. Our suffering does not atone for sin and is only a means of growth—if we use it to learn. We reject "Prosperity Theology," the teaching that God has promised health and wealth to those who obey him.

Death, Dying, and Afterlife

Death is fundamentally about separation. Physical death involves separation of the soul and spirit from the body. Spiritual death is a separation from God, and eternal death is the result of the choice to avoid life in Him. Eternal life is the opposite of eternal death and is focused not only on the length of life after death but on the quality of life that begins when one is reconciled to God through faith in a relationship with Jesus Christ.

Quick and Condensed Definitions of Terms

Word of God or Word—Christian Bible.

New Birth—An infusion of the life of God into individuals the moment they believe. It marks the beginning of eternal life. (*Born again* is a resultant term. So also is *Indwelling of the Spirit*, the life of God, in the third person of the Trinity, coming to permanently reside in the believer.)

Justification—The act of God, who in the event of a person's faith, considers the substitutionary death of Christ as payment for that individual's sin. He is then deemed innocent before God.

The filling of the Spirit—The person who is "filled with the Spirit," has a demeanor that reflects the nature of God. This state is not necessarily constant but varies as the person submits and allows the spirit to "will and do" of His good pleasure.

Signs, wonders, and miracles—Signs may or may not be supernatural but are events that happen to authenticate truth. Thus, the sign "You shall find the Baby, wrapped in swaddling clothes and lying in a manger," is not supernatural but authenticates by its correct prediction. Wonders are awe inspiring, not necessarily miraculous or authenticating, but attention getting. Miracles are events that are against the laws of nature and manifest God's power. They may or may not also be signs or wonders.

Faith—Different kinds exist; some are not saving faith. Faith that is only the expectation and delight in miracles may not be saving faith. Faith where truth does not replace falsehood is not saving faith. Faith involves trusting in the person of Christ to be the true representative of God. It is not just the acceptance of His existence; it also involves trust in His Calvary work alone for our salvation. Faith is not a work, but a resting from our works.

Prayer

Prayer is simply talking to God. It may be praise, thanksgiving, confession, intercession, supplication, or any other conversation. IFCA members pray individually and corporately. We pray as advocates for others, asking for that which the other one needs. A Christian's prayers are always heard. They help the persons praying or prayed for to realize their heart attitude to the One who totally understands us. In prayer for the sick, our primary goal is to articulate that we belong to One who is greater than all our problems and who is interested in our outcomes and, while sharing our feelings, is bent on doing what is really best. The IFCA Christian's ultimate concern is to be like Jesus.

Religious Calendar

One is not to be judged because of observing or not observing certain days. God has specified certain days as special to certain people. The Sabbath observance is designated as a special ordinance between God and His ancient people Israel (e.g., "It is a sign between Me and the sons of Israel forever"). This sign is instructive to the church, but we are not part of that group set apart by it. We hold that promises and commands made between God and Israel belong to that relationship only, unless they are repeated for us. Christians, from early on, celebrated on the first day of the week in memory of Christ's resurrection.

Health-Promoting Practices

We teach abstinence from things that tend to exert inordinate power over us or are not advantageous to us. We condemn the use of tobacco because of its deleterious effects on the body. Alcohol use in itself is not a sin but increases the potential for abuse and disease. It may, in certain cases, have a medicinal effect.

Healing Rituals

Gathering the church elders to anoint with oil and pray for the sick is well regarded as a ritual; it is also a sign of the person's desire to be dependent on God. But physical healing is not a benefit in Christ's atonement and, thus, is not a response to prayer required of God. We believe that all healing comes from God; sometimes, healing is mediated through medical help, and sometimes, it is a direct act of God.

Other Unique Religious Beliefs, Rites, and Practices Related to Health or Illness

We do not practice any other healing rituals except prayer and anointing.

Unique Religious Beliefs, Rites, and Practices Related to Birthing

Every birth should be celebrated and honored as a miracle from God. Therefore, we would stand in opposition to the practice of deliberately ending such a God-given life through abortion practices.

Circumcision, as a religious practice, is a sign of the covenant between God and the Jewish nation and is neither required nor forbidden of Christians in this age. There is no consensus as to whether Jewish Christians should be circumcised.

Baptism does not affect a child's spiritual status. There is no clear example of infant baptism in the Bible, and it is usually argued from silence. Thus, we do not baptize babies.

Unique Religious Beliefs, Rites, or Practices Related to Childrearing

Following the command of Jesus "to let the little children come to Him," IFCA families often place their children under Bible teaching when they are as young as 2 years. Sunday classes are offered for children of all ages, and the Bible is taught on their learning level. There are also weekday opportunities for the memorization of Scripture through organizations such as AWANA (an evangelical organization named from a phrase in 2 Timothy 2:15, Approved Workmen Are Not Ashamed).

All persons must come to saving faith in Christ as individuals. This is not a ritual, or ceremony, but an event between the individual and God. That saving event is to be followed by the ritual of water baptism by immersion. In IFCA churches, baptism is not so much an initiation into membership but a confession of salvation.

Unique Beliefs, Practices, and Rituals Surrounding Dying, Death, and Bereavement

There are no required postmortem practices. It is customary for the local church members to gather to be encouraged by the Word of God at such times. Often it is the choice of the departed or the family that this occasion should be used to publicly explain the meaning of death and the hope of resurrection.

Role of Religious Community (Persons or Organizations) During Health Challenges

IFCA congregations meet on Sundays (often twice) and midweek for prayer. We praise, worship, and teach in these public meetings to encourage one another. Other gatherings are planned to meet special needs. The Lord's Supper, observed during worship services, is a remembrance of our dependence for salvation on Christ's body and shed blood. The elements of the communion neither contain, nor convey grace to the participant, but the remembrance does.

IFCA congregations are free to use any plan for ministry to the sick that is deemed effective and ethical in its environment. Many use ministry plans that originate in parachurch organizations, but none are obliged to do so. The IFCA-wide Chera fellowship cares for the widowed by publishing a magazine devoted to ministering to their needs.

Role of Clergy During Health Challenges

It is considered the obligation of the clergy (typically called Pastor) to visit the sick, widows, and orphans. Most large churches have a designated Visitation Pastor who visits the sick in various institutions and their homes. Some churches assign this role to elected elders.

Unique Religious Aspects of Family Involvement

Most families seek to gather when death seems imminent. It is an important time for ministry as it allows pastoral intervention for the family, including those who express false ideas about death.

Nursing Implications Unique to This Religious Tradition

- IFCA members would typically appreciate a nurse's overt spiritual support, such as offers of prayer or reading comforting Bible passages, and listening carefully to their concerns or fears (e.g., "Why?").

- IFCA members are often comfortable talking about their religious beliefs and may reciprocate the nurse's support by encouraging the nurse to experience saving faith.

- IFCA members honor God as the Creator/Owner of all life; therefore, He has the right to do with His creation as He pleases. He is trustworthy and will, in the end, use all things to bring Himself glory. Nurses can have great confidence as they serve their creator, knowing He is ultimately in control of all things.

- Professing IFCA Christians who are terminal can be encouraged to talk about their anticipation of heaven. The nurse can rejoice with them in the teachings of the Bible concerning heaven and its blessings as a means of true comfort.

FOR MORE INFORMATION

Visit www.ifca.org.
Henry, J. O. (1983). *For such a time as this*. Grandville, MI: IFCA International.
Yancey, P. (1997). *Where is God when it hurts?* Grand Rapids, MI: Zondervan.

EDITOR'S NOTE

*Although IFCA International is a fellowship of non-Pentecostal evangelical independent Bible churches in the United States, IFCA is also a label for a more general movement in the United States made up of many loosely related fellowships of churches. These IFCA churches are independent or denominationally unaffiliated; socially, culturally, and politically conservative; and likewise originated from the movement supporting the Fundamentals. These independent churches are identified sometimes as Bible churches, sometimes as Baptist churches, and other times simply as community churches. The one thing all of these churches (IFCA and IFCA International) have in common is a conservative, orthodox statement of faith essentially rooted in the teachings of the New Testament and the ancient creedal statements of the Christian church. They also all typically place a strong emphasis on a personal conversion experience to Christianity, called being "born again."

16 Jehovah's Witnesses

COMPILERS*:   *Miguel Murillo and Dennis Romain*

Theology and Social History

The modern-day organization of Jehovah's Witnesses (JWs) began toward the end of the 19th century with a small group of Bible students near Pittsburgh, Pennsylvania. The name JWs was adopted in 1931. In 1879, the Bible journal, now called *The Watchtower Announcing Jehovah's Kingdom*, began to be published. It is now published in more than 188 languages and is the world's most widely circulated religious magazine.

Following the model of first-century Christianity, JWs have no clergy–laity division. All baptized members are ordained ministers and share in the preaching and teaching work. Witnesses are organized into congregations of up to 200 members. Spiritually mature men in each congregation serve as elders. A body of elders supervises each congregation. About 20 congregations form a circuit, and about 10 circuits are grouped into a district. Congregations receive periodic visits from traveling elders. Guidance and instructions are provided by a multinational governing body made up of longtime Witnesses who currently serve at the international offices of JWs in Brooklyn, New York. This international brotherhood of people of all races is made up of about 7.5 million practicing members organized into more than 107,000 congregations in more than 236 lands.

JWs respect human laws, except when they contradict Biblical mandates. JW belief and behavior follows directly from their study of the Bible (New World Translation, a translation completed by JW scholars). The admonition found in Acts 15:28–29 to abstain from fornication, blood, and idolatry greatly influences JW behaviors. For example, to abstain from idolatry can mean not having religious or secular icons (e.g., not worshipping a picture of Christ or having a poster of a rock star). Because JWs maintain allegiance to the true God, rather than any national government, they refrain from performing military service, pledging allegiance to a flag or leader, or voting.

Deity/God or Ultimate Other

JWs are monotheistic, believing that Jehovah God is the only true God; Jesus is God's son, a distinct person and part of the creation by God. Jehovah is concerned and cares for all persons individually. One must approach Jehovah God through Jesus Christ on the merits of his ransom sacrifice, which was necessary for redeeming mankind.

Views on Health and Well-Being

JWs want to live long and healthy lives. JW beliefs promote respect for life and help to prevent many common medical problems (e.g., AIDS, hepatitis, and other bloodborne disease). Like anyone else, when JWs are sick, they seek medical care. JWs accept the vast majority of treatments available today. The type of medical treatment selected, however, is a matter of personal choice. For example, agreeing to an organ transplant or organ donation is a personal decision.

Although JWs seek to find effective treatment, they do so only if it adheres to Scriptural principles. For example, JWs are careful to obey the Bible's command to abstain from blood, and they avoid any diagnostic or therapeutic procedure that involves spiritism (i.e., the harmful pursuit of supposedly communicating with the spirits of the dead via a medium, see Ecclesiastes 9:5, 10).

Explanations for Disease and Illness

Adam and Eve, our first human parents, were created with perfectly healthy bodies. They were designed to live on earth forever. It was not until they willfully rebelled against God that their bodies became susceptible to disease. By rejecting God's authority, they severed their ties with the Creator, the Source of their perfect life. They became defective. As a result, they got sick and died, just as God had warned them they would. After their rebellion, Adam and Eve could only pass on imperfection to their children (Genesis 1–3, Deuteronomy 32:4, Romans 5:12).

The Nature of Suffering and How to Address It

Suffering is explained in large part to mankind's rejection of God as Ruler, not wanting to submit to his righteous laws and principles. Humans have unwittingly submitted to God's Adversary, Satan. Satan is evil, hateful, deceptive, and cruel. So we should expect the world to reflect the personality of its ruler.

Human imperfection is another reason for the suffering we experience. Sinful humans tend to struggle for dominance, and that often results in wars, oppression, and suffering. A further reason for suffering is "time and unforeseen occurrence" (Ecclesiastes 9:11). People often experience calamity because they are in the wrong place at the wrong time.

Death, Dying, and Afterlife

Death is the cessation of all functions of life, hence, the opposite of life. In the Bible, both humans and animals are spoken of as "expiring," that is, "breathing out" the breath of life. Scriptures also show that death in humans and animals follows the loss of the spirit (active force) of life (see Genesis 6:17, 7:15, 21–22; Ecclesiastes 3:19). Although the vital importance of breathing and of the blood in maintaining the active life force in the body cells is evident, at the same time it is also clear that it is not the cessation of breathing or of heartbeat alone but the disappearance of the life force or spirit from the body cells that brings death as referred to in the Scriptures. The Bible does not require extraordinary measures to be taken to sustain a person if this would merely prolong the dying process.

A knowledge of God's provision of Jesus Christ, who gave himself "a ransom in exchange for many" (Matthew 20:28), is the only means through which humans can be restored to full spiritual as well as physical wholeness. Jesus is able to regenerate mankind, thus giving life to those who exercise faith and are obedient. JWs believe in a resurrection of the dead to life. They look forward to God's Kingdom, the "city having real foundations" (Hebrews 11:10). Jesus' parable in Luke 19:11–27 shows what the "coming of the Kingdom" means: it is coming to execute judgment, to destroy all opposition, and to bring relief and reward to those hoping in it.

Quick and Condensed Definitions of Terms

Jehovah—The personal name of the true God (Isaiah 42:8).

God's Kingdom—An established heavenly government that is soon to come to rule over the earth.

The anointed—Spirit-begotten members who privately know they are going to rule as kings and priests in the heavenly Kingdom to come.

Prayer

True prayer is worshipful address to the true God Jehovah. Prayer involves devotion, trust, respect, and a sense of dependence on the one to whom the prayer is directed. Prayers can involve confession, petitions or requests, expressions of praise and thanksgiving, and vows. Although JWs do not believe in faith healing, they do pray for oneself and others for the strength to overcome difficulty and remain faithful to God.

Religious Calendar

The Memorial (or Lord's Evening Meal) is the most important meeting of the year and calls special attention to the significance of the death of Jesus Christ. It is observed on Nisan 14 (of the Jewish calendar, the time of Passover) during a service in Kingdom Halls. Although JWs believe in the birth and resurrection of Jesus, they do not celebrate Christmas and Easter in contemporary tradition reflective of pagan culture.

Health-Promoting Practices

JWs promote health among believers by offering health education and Bible-based teachings that prevent many health problems. The international monthly magazine *Awake!*, published by JWs, frequently features articles on health and medicine. Although *Awake!* does not dispense medical advice or endorse specific treatments, it does offer up-to-date, accurate information on many health issues. Because it is published in 83 languages with a circulation of more than 36 million copies, *Awake!* often reaches readers who otherwise have limited access to health care or health education. Lifestyle teachings of the religion include the forbidding of tobacco and abuse of drugs. JWs may use alcoholic beverages in moderation but are to avoid drunkenness. JWs closely adhere to the Bible's teaching that sexual relations should be limited to one's marriage partner and shun activities that risk human life. JWs also teach high standards of cleanliness.

Healing Rituals

JWs do not believe in faith healing as practiced today. Jesus and his apostles performed miraculous healings, but these were first-century phenomena and not an ongoing feature of Christianity (1 Corinthians 13:8).

Other Unique Religious Beliefs, Rites, and Practices Related to Health or Illness

JWs refuse blood transfusions because they follow the Bible command to "abstain from . . . blood" (Acts 15:20, 29 and Acts 21:25 as well as Genesis 9:3–4, Leviticus 7:26, 27; 17:1, 2, 10–12; Deuteronomy 12:23–25). JWs request the use of nonblood medical alternatives, which are widely accepted and used by the medical community. Given that the Bible makes no clear statement about the use of minor blood fractions or the immediate reinfusion of a patient's own blood during surgery, the use of such treatments is a matter of personal choice. JWs accept reliable nonblood medical alternatives, medicines, and surgical techniques used in place of blood transfusion. JWs do not accept whole blood transfusions or any of the primary components of blood, red cells, white cells, platelets, or plasma. Individuals may accept fractions of those components (e.g., hemoglobin, interferons, clotting factors, albumin), based on their own conscientious decision. JWs do not accept preoperative autologous blood donation. Autotransfusion techniques such as hemodilution and cell salvage are a matter for personal decision. Likewise, use of a heart–lung machine primed with nonblood fluids, hemodialysis without a blood prime, and hemodilution are all for the JW patient to conscientiously decide. Likewise, some Witness patients accept tests in which a quantity of blood is withdrawn in order to tag or mix it with medicine and then reinfuse it.

Although the Bible specifically forbids consuming blood, no Biblical command pointedly forbids the taking in of tissue or bone from another human. Therefore, whether to accept an organ transplant is a personal medical decision.

JWs have no objection to vaccines, in general. Some vaccines contain minor blood fractions, and use of these is a matter of personal choice.

Although health care settings typically dispose of all biological products (body wastes, diseased tissues, blood) after they have been analyzed, if a JW patient had valid reason to doubt that such normal practice was going to be followed, he or she would, for religious reasons, want all such products disposed.

Although moderate use of alcohol is acceptable, Scriptural principles of moderation and respect for one's life and mental faculties would rule out substance abuse (e.g., tobacco and recreational drugs). The medical use of drugs, including narcotics for severe pain, under the supervision of a physician, is a personal matter.

JWs are required to abstain from eating blood and the meat of animals from which blood has not been properly drained. Aside from this Bible injunction, there is no restriction on what is to be eaten. Because abattoirs typically drain blood from meat, and traces of blood in meat is acceptable, no special meats or diets are necessary.

Unique Religious Beliefs, Rites, and Practices Related to Birthing

If a birthing setting is likely to save a placenta and umbilical cord for blood extraction, a JW mother would request that her placenta and umbilical cord be disposed and not used in any way.

JWs leave the choice of male circumcision for parents to make. Female circumcision is unreasonable mutilation.

Life begins at conception. Deliberately induced abortion is viewed as the willful taking of human life. If, at the time of childbirth, a choice must be made between the life of the mother and that of the child, it is up to the individuals concerned to make that decision. Witnesses avoid contraceptive methods that are abortive.

JWs view in vitro fertilization involving the egg and sperm from persons who are not married to each other as comparable to adultery and thus unacceptable. Gestational surrogacy is also considered to be unacceptable.

Unique Religious Beliefs, Rites, or Practices Related to Childrearing

Families are encouraged to have 20–60 min of "family worship" once a week at a time of their choice. During this time, usually a night during the week, the father (or mother if she is a solo parent) will lead a Bible-based discussion on a topic pertinent to the children (e.g., manners, dating).

Discipline in the sense of instruction, training, and loving correction is vital in molding the lives of young children. Child neglect or abuse has no justification.

Unique Beliefs, Practices, and Rituals Surrounding Dying, Death, and Bereavement

JWs reject the belief in the immortality of the soul. Rather, they believe that death is like sleep, and the deceased await a resurrection. The dead are in God's memorial tombs (i.e., God's memory). Thus, JWs reject notions like the dead becoming ghosts or angels. JWs are buried or cremated following the customs of their local culture, as long as these do not conflict with Bible teaching. For example, if in the deceased's culture there is a way in which flowers are used at a funeral or at a grave site that has a false religious meaning locally, JWs would avoid that.

Role of Religious Community (Persons or Organizations) During Health Challenges

JWs meet regularly twice a week (e.g., Sunday and Tuesday evening) in meeting places called Kingdom Halls. They are also encouraged to have family worship once a weeknight weekly. Their meetings, which are open to the public, are essentially Bible studies, allowing for audience participation. One of the weekly meetings, the Theocratic Ministry School, helps congregation members develop teaching, reading, and research skills. Another is a 30-min Bible discourse, which is normally followed by a study of the Bible by means of the *Watchtower* magazine. Meetings begin and end with song and prayer, and there is no solicitation of funds. When members of a congregation are not able to attend such meetings because of infirmity or other limiting circumstances, there may be certain provisions for them to listen into the meetings via telephone or recorded media. JWs also gather in larger assemblies twice a year (by the hundreds) and conventions once a year (by the thousands).

Although each congregation does not have a formal organized ministry for the sick, most large, urban areas worldwide have a Hospital Liaison Committee (HLC). These HLCs are comprised of elders well-educated in what JWs will accept or refuse as medical treatment and work to assist communication between JW patients and health care professionals. For instance, they can provide information on alternative medical care based on the latest medical research to primary care physicians or to emergency department staff.

Also available to JW patients and families are Patient Visitation Group members. These elders provide pastoral care at hospitals and can contact the HLC when necessary. They often provide assistance such as help finding accommodation for family members of hospitalized patients or transportation to Kingdom Hall meetings.

Role of Clergy During Health Challenges

As there is no clergy–laity distinction, congregation elders take the lead in helping those that need help (see above); this help is primarily spiritual support but may also include material help. Members of a congregation also offer support and encouragement to members in need.

Unique Religious Aspects of Family Involvement

If a JW patient has a family who are not JW, disagreement can occur between them regarding whether to accept a blood transfusion. Most JWs have a durable power of attorney, which states the patient's instructions about therapeutics, and this legal document should be respected. The majority will carry on their person a wallet-sized identity card, which states their refusal of blood.

Nursing Implications Unique to This Religious Tradition

- Any practice that JWs perceive as conflicting with Biblical truth or have a meaning based on religious error are avoided. However, they recognize that all kinds of objects, designs, and practices have, at some time or place, been given a false interpretation or have been linked with unscriptural teachings. (For example, in the past, trees have been worshiped, the heart shape has been viewed as sacred, and incense has been used in pagan ceremonies.) Thus, a JW makes a decision about what to do considering what the customs are in his or her contemporary society. If a current custom has a false religious meaning (e.g., a cross, Halloween), then it is avoided. JWs would thus not send flowers in the form of a cross or a red heart if that is viewed as having religious significance. That is not to say, though, that simply providing a bouquet at a funeral or giving flowers to a friend in the hospital must be viewed as a religious act that must be avoided.

- JWs reject blood transfusions (see above, *Other unique religious beliefs, rites, and practices*). To infuse blood without a JW's permission is akin to medical rape. JWs carry on their person an Advance Medical Directive/Release document that directs that no blood transfusions be given under any circumstances and releasing health care personnel and institutions from responsibility for any damages caused by the refusal of blood. When entering the hospital, release forms should be signed that state matters similarly and deal more specifically with the needed hospital care.

- JWs prefer to use their own New World translation of the Bible. If a patient wanted a nurse to read a Biblical passage, it is best read from this translation. Other mainstream translations, however, are acceptable if a New World Translation is not available.

- Many hospitalized JWs will choose not to have any chaplain visit them for fear that this may involve some other religious organization. Clarify if they want a visit from their elders or simply someone from their congregation.

FOR MORE INFORMATION

Visit http://www.jw-media.org/ or http://www.jw.org or http://www.watchtower.org/

What does the Bible really teach? (2005). Brooklyn, NY: Watchtower Bible and Tract Society of New York.

NOTE

*This information was compiled from material found at http://www.jw-media.org and http://www.watchtower.org, as well as in the *Watchtower* and *Awake!* magazines.

17 Jews

CONTRIBUTOR: *Rabbi Elliot N. Dorff, PhD*

NURSE REVIEWER: *Eileen Schonfeld, BS ED, RN*

Theology and Social History

Tracing its roots to Abraham and Sarah (c. 1700 BCE or BC), the Jewish
tradition produced the Torah (the Five Books of Moses or Pentateuch) as
well as the rest of the Hebrew Bible. A long rabbinic tradition of interpretation, expansion, and application of the Bible occurred in books such
as the Mishnah (oral tradition after the Bible), the Talmud (amplification
of the Mishnah), Midrash, legal codes, rabbinic rulings on specific cases,
philosophy, literature, and more. The Jewish tradition places strong em-
phases on family, community, education, and repairing the world (*Tikkun
Olam*), with a very strong sense of moral mission and yet a deep tolerance
for pluralism. It encourages discussion, debate, and questions. Indeed, every page of the Talmud is one debate after another. That feisty quality is
prized by Jews.

The homeland of the Jewish people is Israel, the land promised by
God to Abraham, Isaac, and Jacob. It is the land to which Moses led the
Israelites after their slavery in Egypt. Since the destruction of the First
Temple in 586 BCE, however, Jews have lived all over the world. Currently
numbering a little over 13 million, Jews constitute only 0.2% of the world's
population. Although the largest Jewish community is in the United States
(about 5.5 million), 5 million live in Israel. Jewish communities numbering in the hundreds of thousands live in Australia, the United Kingdom,
France, Russia, and Argentina.

Because of the strong sense of communal ties and traditions, many
Jews—as many as half in the United States—identify as secular Jews.
Among religiously affiliated Jews in the United States, going from most to
least traditional in practice and belief, about 20% are Orthodox, 33% are
Conservative, 2% are Reconstructionist, 38% are Reform, and the rest in-
clude Renewal and "just Jewish" (i.e., without any movement affiliation).

Deity/God or Ultimate Other

Judaism is theistic. It is often characterized as "ethical monotheism."
That is, it asserts that God is moral and demands morality of us. Most
Jewish theologies that have been written over the ages depict God in

personal terms: God loves, commands, enters into a Covenant with the People Israel and another Covenant with all Children of Noah, and so forth. A small number of Jewish theologies are deistic, picturing God as the Creative Force that created the world and continues to influence us, or as the Process of creation. Either way, God is definitely involved in human lives. Jews communicate with God by studying and practicing God's laws as interpreted in the tradition, by prayer, and by acting to improve the lives of people and repairing the world (*Tikkun Olam*).

Views on Health and Well-Being

Health and well-being include not only physical health, but mental and emotional health as well. In Genesis, we read "it is not good for a man to live alone" (Genesis 2:18), and Judaism emphasizes the importance not only of marriage but also of strong ties to the community, for "all Jews are responsible for each other" (Talmud, *Shevu'ot* 39a). This leads to the Jewish duty (*mitzvah* or commandment) to visit the sick (*bikkur holim*) for the tradition understands that well-being, perhaps especially when one is sick, requires companionship. The tradition also understands that age changes one's state of health (e.g., see the description of old age in Ecclesiastes 12). At any age, though, we each have a duty to take care of our health because our body belongs to God, as does everything else (e.g., Deuteronomy 10:14). We have a sacred duty to maintain God's property through good eating, sleep, hygiene, exercise, and following physicians' orders when we get sick.

Explanations for Disease and Illness

Although Deuteronomy links illness to sin (e.g., 28:15, 21–22, 27–28), Job disputes this linkage. Ancient sources, of course, did not know about microorganisms, so they explained diseases in terms of disobeying God. Evidence shows otherwise now. Because some of the things people do (e.g., eat too much, smoke, avoid exercise) do raise the probability that they will get sick, Jews have a duty to avoid such behaviors. Some illnesses, though, are no fault of one's own. They are caused by one's genes, a virus, or other factors over which one has no control. Jews are to take care of their health to the extent that they can, but they should also realize that many diseases just happen, regardless of one's health behaviors, morality, or piety.

The Nature of Suffering and How to Address It

Jewish tradition posits that the prevention and alleviation of suffering is a duty. For example, if one assaults another, one of the remedies that the assailant must pay is for the pain and suffering he or she caused the victim (Mishnah, *Bava Kamma* 8:1). Suffering is *not* a punishment from God or the price for a better life after death. Instead, the real meaning of suffering is twofold. Meaning is found first in what that person gains in wisdom and coping skills and, second, in what the person's caring community—family, friends, health care providers, and others—do to prevent or alleviate it. Suffering, in other words, invokes a duty in the sufferer's community to act like the caring community that they should be.

Death, Dying, and Afterlife

Jewish tradition defines death as the cessation of heartbeat and breath. Once the Harvard criteria were formulated in the 1960s, most rabbis accepted whole brain death, including the brain stem, as the equivalent of the traditional markers. Some ultra-Orthodox Jews, however, do not accept this definition.

Jewish tradition supports belief in an afterlife. Given that nobody has been there and come back to tell us what it is like, rabbis, in describing it, wrote their fondest wishes large (e.g., in the afterlife, one does not have to work for a living, the days are spent studying Torah with God as teacher). The primary reason that the rabbis of the Mishnah, Talmud, and Midrash believed in an afterlife and why some Jews do today is to reconcile with God's justice the fact that "the righteous suffer, and the evil prosper" (Talmud, *Berakhot* 7a). The biblical phrase used for death is that people are "gathered to their ancestors" (Judges 2:9), so presumably, one reconnects with one's deceased family in an afterlife.

Quick and Condensed Definitions of Terms

Bikkur Holim—The sacred duty to visit the sick.

Kaddish—The prayer affirming God's holiness and might that is used also for mourners (see "Unique Beliefs, Practices, and Rituals Surrounding Dying, Death, and Bereavement"; see also "Prayer").

Kashrut—The practice of "keeping kosher," observing the Jewish dietary rules (see *Nursing Implications*).

Mitzvah—Commandment or sacred obligation.

Viddui—Jewish confessional prayer.

She'ma—Watchword prayer of the Jewish faith: "Hear o Israel, the Lord our God, the Lord is One."

Prayer

Prayer is an important part of the Jewish tradition. Traditional Jews pray three times a day. Ideally, Jewish prayers are said in the presence of a *minyan*, a prayer quorum consisting of at least 10 Jews 13 years of age or older (in Orthodox circles, they must be males), and some prayers are said only when part of a *minyan*, but most Jewish prayers can be said individually, too.

Any Jew may pray for any other Jew (or non-Jew, for that matter), and religious leaders (i.e., rabbis, cantors) may pray for any Jew or non-Jew as well. Prayers for the ill can be said in the presence of the sick person or elsewhere. *Mi shebarakh*, the beginning words of the prayer for the sick, petitions: "May He who blessed our ancestors . . . bless this sick person [followed by the name]." Prayers for the ill are commonly recited during synagogue services, especially on the Sabbath, in part to pray for the recovery of the people mentioned and in part to announce to the community that someone is ill so that they will know and visit them.

Religious Calendar

Shabbat (or, in Yiddish, "Shabbes") is the Sabbath, which takes place between 18 min before sunset on Friday to about 40 min after sunset on Saturday. During the Sabbath, traditional Jews do not do a variety of activities. For example, they may not write, do business, cook, do laundry, and some do not use electricity either. *Shabbat* can include worship in the synagogue on Friday evenings, Saturday mornings, and Saturday afternoons, as well as family meals on Friday evening and Saturday at lunch, to which guests are often invited, and there is a lot of conversation and singing.

Similar restrictions apply to the three pilgrimage festivals of *Pesah* (Passover), *Shavu'ot* (the Feast of Weeks), and *Sukkot* (the Feast of Tabernacles), as well as the High Holy Days (Rosh Hashanah [Jewish New Year] and Yom Kippur [Day of Atonement]). On the first two nights of Passover, families have a *Seder*, a meal that allows the retelling of the Exodus. During Passover, no leavened foods are eaten; many other foods are proscribed and prescribed. On Yom Kippur, Jews fast from sunset to sunset. (These rules are set aside, however, if the patient's doctor says that he or she must eat or must eat certain foods.) The High Holy Days mark a 10-day period in which Jews do a "soul accounting," and ask for forgiveness from other people and from God. They are prompted by the liturgy to think about the big questions of life and how they can do better next year.

The Jewish calendar is based on a lunar calendar, and so although Passover always occurs in March or early April, *Shavu'ot* in late May or early June, and High Holy Days and *Sukkot* in September or October, the exact dates of holidays will vary from year to year. Look at a Jewish calendar to determine when these fall in any given year. In addition, there are several popular minor holidays; "minor" in that they are not mentioned in the Torah and do not have the same strictures that Torah festivals do.

These include Hanukkah, Purim, Israel's Day of Independence, and Tisha B'Av.

Health-Promoting Practices

The dietary laws ("keeping kosher") are not intended for the purposes of health. One can follow them and eat very badly from the standpoint of health. They do, however, encourage Jews to focus on what they are eating. Washing oneself at least once a week on Friday in honor of the approaching Sabbath, as well as after menses, was common practice long before anyone knew about the needs of hygiene. (Traditionally, the washing after menses occurred—and still does for more traditional Jews—at the *mikvah*, a pool that has running water from a fresh source.) Similarly, the Jewish ritual requirement to wash one's hands before a meal may have warded off some illnesses during the Middle Ages and to this day.

More directly influencing health promotion among Jews is the belief that one's body belongs to God; therefore, one has a sacred responsibility to take care of it and to avoid unnecessary dangers (e.g., smoking, alcohol abuse). Likewise, Jews have historically honored physicians, and this has set the foundation for Jews to be interested in promoting their own health and that of others.

Healing Rituals

The *Mi shebarakh* prayer (see "Prayer") is commonly requested, and usually, it is a knowledgeable Jew who recites it. Anyone's prayer in any language, though, that asks for healing or comfort will be appreciated by a Jewish patient who requests it. Anyone can also read from the Book of Psalms with the patient.

Other Unique Religious Beliefs, Rites, and Practices Related to Health or Illness

Some Jews, especially older ones or those from the Orient, may be superstitious and observe some different practices. A common one is to tie a red ribbon around the bedpost to ward off evil spirits. Another is to put one of the psalms on the headboard to invoke the presence of God.

Unique Religious Beliefs, Rites, and Practices Related to Birthing

Jews circumcise their sons on the eighth day after birth (the child's *brit milah*, Covenant of circumcision, or "bris"). This typically is done in the parents' home or synagogue, but it can be done anywhere, including a hospital. If the child is judged by a pediatrician not to be healthy enough to be circumcised on the eighth day, then the circumcision is postponed until he is healthy enough to have it done. The circumcision is accompanied by a specific liturgy; it is not the medical procedure alone. There is no such ritual for daughters in traditional Jewish practice, but since the 1970s, parents have been creating rituals of their own, often involving pouring a bit of water on the child's feet. Traditionally, sons are named as part of the liturgy of the *brit milah*, and daughters are named in the synagogue during a Sabbath morning service.

Unique Religious Beliefs, Rites, or Practices Related to Childrearing

Another important rite of passage is the Bar/Bat (male/female) Mitzvah ("son/daughter of the commandments"). Usually during the child's 12th or 13th year, they read all or part of the Torah portion for the week and lead the worship service. That brings them into full participation as an "adult" within the faith.

Unique Beliefs, Practices, and Rituals Surrounding Dying, Death, and Bereavement

When death is near, there are prayers that Jews do for themselves or others do for them: These include the *tzidduk ha-din* (accepting God's justice) and the *viddui* (the Jewish confessional asking for forgiveness). Once the person has died, the person's eyes are closed. In Orthodox and Conservative Jewish communities, where a holy community or *hevrah kaddishah* exists, it should be called to care for the body. Because Jews respect modesty even in death, this group (of men if the deceased was male, women if the deceased was female) wash the body first for hygienic reasons and then for ritual reasons and then clothe it in linen shrouds. Someone stays with the body overnight, usually reciting passages from the Book of Psalms. The body is buried the next day in a closed, plain wooden casket. If relatives need to fly in from out of town, or if the Sabbath or one of the Torah's holidays intervenes, the burial is postponed, but usually not for more than a day or two. Jewish law does not allow cremation, but some Reform or secular Jews do cremate, and then some bury the cremains.

At the funeral, the rabbi and, often, relatives and friends speak about the deceased. They will recite a few psalms and *el maleh rahamim*, "God who is full of mercy," a prayer that asks God to give a proper and honored rest to the deceased. The funeral usually happens in a room at the cemetery, but for people who were very active in the Jewish community, where a large audience is anticipated, the funeral may take place in the synagogue. The body is then brought to the grave and buried, with those present shoveling three shovelfuls of dirt into the grave. Then, the family recites the *kaddish*.

Traditionally, the next 7 days are the period of *shivah* ("seven"); however, now, this is often 3–5 days. During *shivah*, family and friends go to the home of the mourners for morning, afternoon, and evening services (to make a *minyan* there), and people bring food and take care of the other daily needs of the family. People are supposed to come during the day to help the mourners remember their loved one, often by asking questions of the mourner or by telling their own stories about the deceased. The mourners are not supposed to go to work during *shivah*. They sit on low stools to symbolize their low emotional state and cover mirrors to refrain from thinking about themselves. The visiting and reminiscing does not officially take place on the Sabbath, but the day counts toward the seven. The last morning of *shivah*, after services, those gathered may accompany the mourners for a walk around the block, symbolizing their reentry into normal life. During the first month after the burial, the siblings, parents, and spouse of the deceased recite the *kaddish* prayer in the synagogue services morning and evening; some do it for longer periods of time. Children recite *kaddish* for their parents in the synagogue morning and evening for 11 months. After that, people recite that prayer on the anniversary of their relative's death. More orthodox men do not shave during *shivah* and, when mourning for a parent, for the first 30 days after the funeral. In modern times, some families (especially Reform Jews) do only part of these rituals.

Role of Religious Community (Persons or Organizations) During Health Challenges

Some Jews gather for prayer in the synagogue each morning and evening (around sunset) to recite prayers. More attend the synagogue on Sabbaths and festivals. Jews also gather in synagogues for classes and other educational and cultural activities, social events, life cycle ceremonies, and social action work.

Some communities still have Jewish hospitals, where access to kosher food and Jewish chaplains and worship are more likely. Most communities have a Jewish home for the aging, and some have assisted living facilities under Jewish auspices that offer kosher food and worship and educational activities. Jewish Family Service exists in most Jewish communities, and it offers counseling and a variety of other services to those with mental health needs, including some that are directly related to a person's physical health (e.g., addiction programs, exercise programs for seniors).

Many synagogues have established a *Bikkur Holim* group, who learn how best to visit patients and who take it upon themselves to do that regularly. Some synagogues also ask their teens to visit homebound people on a regular basis as part of their social service work. Jewish Family Service in some communities sponsors similar groups.

Role of Clergy During Health Challenges

Congregational rabbis and cantors, as well as specially trained volunteers, regularly see it as part of their duties to visit the sick, especially those in hospitals and nursing homes.

Unique Religious Aspects of Family Involvement

The rabbis interpreted the biblical commandment "Honor your father and mother" to require adult children to feed their parents when they cannot feed themselves and to assist them in walking when they cannot do that on their own. The rabbis saw personal service to one's parents as the ideal. This was the practice until two generations ago, for people lived in extended family configurations. In contemporary society, however, where people live in nuclear families and where both members of a couple often work during the day and therefore cannot attend to elderly parents for much of the week, this is much less common. Often elderly parents live on their own for as long as possible and then in assisted living facilities. Children and grandchildren, however, see it as their duty to visit as often as possible and to make sure that their parents are well treated.

Nursing Implications Unique to This Religious Tradition

- *Kashrut*, or keeping kosher, means that a Jew may eat only animals that have split hooves and chew their cud, fish that have fins and scales, and domesticated fowl; meat from animals slaughtered in a particular way to avoid pain to the animal; and meat that has had the blood drained out. Also, *Kashrut* proscribes that meat and milk products may not be cooked, served, or eaten together. Some Jews who keep kosher will require specially certified kosher meals for all their meals, whereas others will require that only for meat and fowl (where the restrictions are greater) but will be satisfied with dairy or fish meals without certification of their kosher status. If a kosher meal is not available, a vegan meal will suffice. These dietary rules are observed by the more orthodox and traditional Jew.

- In some settings, nurses may assist patients in knowing about Jewish worship opportunities in the facility and in getting them there. The same applies to holiday celebrations or observances. Sometimes just a little thing may mean a lot. It is traditional, for example, to eat slices of apple dipped in honey on Rosh Hashanah, symbolic of hope for a sweet new year. Simply supplying that to a Jewish patient at that time, if permissible, can be meaningful. Patients on special diets can have this altered (e.g., eat applesauce or dip apple slices in artificially sweetened maple syrup). Similarly, it is customary for Jews (especially women) to light two candles 18 min (or earlier) before sunset to mark the onset of the Sabbath, a Festival, or High Holy Day. Arranging for that in a fire-safe place (e.g., electric or battery operated candles) can restore a sense of normalcy and connectedness for a Jewish patient.

- For Jews in a health care institution on *Shabbat* or other major holy day, consult with them about how to restore a sense of *Shabbat*. They may want uninterrupted time for prayers, or they may want to not interrupt therapies that speed their healing.

- For the dying patient, make sure *tzidduk ha-din* and *viddui* prayers are offered prior to death. When the patient has died, close the eyelids, follow your institution's protocol for postmortem care, and if desired by the family and if possible, call the *hevrah kaddishah*. (Ideally, this is arranged with the family or leaders of a local synagogue.) Avoid leaving the body unattended until this group arrives.

- If a Jewish patient asks a non-Jewish nurse for prayer, the nurse can inquire as to how the patient prefers to address the Divine. Of course, addressing the prayer to Allah or Jesus would be insensitive! Labeling the Divine "God" or "Lord" would be acceptable.

FOR MORE INFORMATION

Dorff, E. N. (1998). *Matters of life and death: A Jewish approach to modern medical ethics.* Philadelphia, PA: Jewish Publishing Society.

Jacobs, L. (1984). *The book of Jewish belief.* West Orange, NJ: Behrman House.

Jacobs, L. (1987). *The book of Jewish practice.* West Orange, NJ: Behrman House.

Kushner, H. S. (1993). *To life! A celebration of Jewish being and thinking.* Boston, MA: Little Brown.

18 Latter-Day Saints (Mormons)

CONTRIBUTORS: *Brent L. Top, PhD, and Lieutenant Justin B. Top*

NURSE REVIEWER: *Lynn Callister, PhD, RN, FAAN*

Theology and Social History

The Church of Jesus Christ of Latter-Day Saints (LDS) was organized in upstate New York in 1830 with Joseph Smith, Jr. as its first president and prophet. Although a Christian faith tradition, the Church is neither Catholic, Orthodox, nor Protestant by origin. Rather, the Church views itself as a restoration of primitive Christianity. LDS believe that Christ's original Church, including the fullness of His gospel teachings and the power and authority He conferred upon the apostles, was corrupted over time, and lost from the earth. This restoration came about through a series of heavenly manifestations to Joseph Smith in response to his earnest prayers to know which church he should join. Joseph Smith claimed that God the Father and Jesus Christ appeared to him and instructed him not to join any church for all of them, though each possessed remnants of the truth, lacked priesthood authority and the fullness of the gospel. In time, God restored His priesthood to Joseph Smith and others by the means of heavenly messengers. In addition, truths that had been lost from the earth during centuries of apostasy were again restored through the latter-day prophet, Joseph Smith. These restorative revelations included additional scripture, *The Book of Mormon: Another Testament of Jesus Christ*. Smith claimed that an angel appeared to him and showed him where ancient gold plates were hidden and instructed him to translate them by the power of God that would be given to him. Smith taught that the plates contained a spiritual record of God's people on the American continent written by ancient prophets—a companion record to the Bible, the spiritual record of God's people in the Old World.

Persecuted because of their beliefs, practices, and claims of heavenly manifestations, members of the Church were forced to move from New York to Ohio and eventually to Missouri. Mormons were ultimately compelled to leave the state of Missouri or be "exterminated" by order of the governor. They established themselves in Nauvoo, Illinois, where they lived in relative peace until Joseph Smith was murdered in 1844. Brigham Young then became the leader of the Church and prepared them to move to the Great Basin of western America in what is one of the largest pioneer migrations in the U.S. history. Arriving in 1847 in the Salt Lake valley, the Mormons quickly established thriving communities throughout the inter-mountain area of what would become the states of Utah, Idaho, Arizona, Nevada, and California. Although the Church today is among the larg-est Christian denominations in the United States, it has more members outside of the United States. With a membership of over 14 million, the LDS church has nearly 30,000 congregations found in over 130 countries throughout the world.

Deity/God or Ultimate Other

The first article of faith for LDS is: "We believe in God the Eternal Father and in His son Jesus Christ and in the Holy Ghost." Like other Christians, LDS believe that God, as the universal father of mankind, is indeed con-cerned for the well-being of each individual. We can communicate with God through sincere prayer.

Views on Health and Well-Being

LDS believe that every human being is both a physical being and a spiri-tual being. The human body is a "temple of God" (see 1 Corinthians 3:17; 2 Corinthians 6:16)—meaning that it is the earthly "tabernacle" for the immortal spiritual essence of man. The physical body is essential to God's spiritual purposes for man both now and in eternity. Therefore, LDS rec-ognize that true health is a combination of physical, emotional, and spiri-tual factors, and each is interconnected with the others. Not taking proper care of one's physical health also affects one's spiritual and emotional well-being and vice versa. Thus, striving to take care of one's physical health through proper nutrition and hygiene, exercise, and sound medical practices is a spiritual duty.

LDS adhere to a distinctive health code known as the "Word of Wisdom," which prohibits the use of tobacco, alcohol, tea, coffee, and harmful, habit-forming drugs. In addition, this health code that Mormons believe was given to the church in 1833 via divine revelation to Joseph Smith, advocates consumption of meat "sparingly," and that grains, fruits, and vegetables are "good for the food of man" (Doctrine and Covenants 89:12–17). To LDS, the Word of Wisdom is a health code for both the body and the spirit, with the promise of both improved health and spiritual well-being. Spiritual health to LDS would be akin to what the New Testament calls the "fruit of the Spirit"—love, joy, peace, long suffering, gentleness, goodness, faith, meekness, and self-control (see Galatians 5:22–23).

Explanations for Disease and Illness

LDS reject the notion that suffering is punishment from God. Without rejecting or minimizing the role that God has in individual lives, LDS teach that disease, pain, problems, and suffering can be traced to two main sources: (1) free will (or agency) and (2) nature. A fundamental LDS teaching is that next to the bestowal of life, freedom of choice is God's greatest earthly gift to man. Yet, choices also have consequences. As a result, sickness or suffering can come as consequences of our own choices (e.g., choosing not to exercise or eat healthfully causing heart disease or diabetes) as well as from the choices of others (e.g., victim of second-hand smoke). Free will—whether our own choices or the choices of those around us—is like a two-edged sword. It can produce positive or negative consequence—depending upon the choice.

A second major explanation for disease and sickness would be the fundamental laws of nature. LDS believe that even though God is author of those laws, He allows those laws to operate freely in our lives on earth. Like freewill, this can lead to both positive and negative results. Genetics, for example, may be the reason why one person may be more prone to disease and sickness and another less prone. The laws of nature tend to be indiscriminate—good people get sick and die and so do the less righteous. Jesus taught "That ye may be the children of your Father which is in heaven: for he maketh his sun to rise on the evil and the good, and sendeth rain on the just and on the unjust" (Holy Bible, Matthew 5:45).

From the fall of Adam and Eve in the Garden of Eden, sickness, disease, pain, and suffering have been inherent in the world. Because we live in a fallen world as fallen creatures, we, in a way, begin to die the moment we are born. Although we are commanded to take care of the bodies we have been given, aging, sickness and death are part of God's plan.

The Nature of Suffering and How to Address It

Although God does not personally cause every sickness, accident, or painful problem in life, LDS believe that God can and does use suffering for the good of the individual. We believe that whatever the cause of suffering and however painful it is, God can turn it to good. Suffering need not be senseless. It can promote spiritual growth, sanctify and refine one's life, and strengthen one's relationship with God and others. As one LDS leader taught, "No pain that we suffer, no trial that we experience is wasted. It ministers to our education, to the development of such qualities as patience, faith, fortitude and humility. All that we suffer and all that we endure, especially when we endure it patiently, builds up our characters, purifies our hearts, expands our souls, and makes us more tender and charitable, more worthy to be called the children of God." Because LDS believe that this life is a time for men to prepare to meet God and dwell with Him eternally, it is believed that often the suffering and trials one encounters in life are part of the preparation for eternal life. Lessons one learns and character traits one develops through exposure to and faithful endurance of the pains and problems of life go with us into the next life and will be to our advantage in the eternities. Despite the good that can come through facing pain with courage and faith, LDS do not seek for such suffering but accept it as part of God's plan and strive to learn and grow from it.

Death, Dying, and Afterlife

Prior to our birth on earth, we lived as spirit sons and daughters of God. Thus, earth life is what could be viewed as the second act of a three act play. Death of the physical body is like the closing of the curtain on that act. The immortal spirit, like a hand removed from a glove, separates from the body and is "taken home to that God who gave [it] life" (Book of Mormon, Alma 40:11; see also Holy Bible, Ecclesiastes 12:7). LDS believe that because of the Fall of Adam all mankind will die a physical death, and because of Christ's redemptive power over death, all will likewise be resurrected from death. LDS believe in a literal and universal resurrection. The Book of Mormon likewise teaches that "the spirit and the body shall be reunited again in its perfect form" (Alma 11:42–43).

LDS canon and doctrinal teachings of Church leaders, whom Mormons accept as modern-day prophets and revelators, declare that after death, the spirits of all people enter into a realm or existence to await the universal resurrection—the ultimate reuniting of the spirit and body. This temporary abode is called the spirit world. It is a place where the departed may "rest from all their troubles and from all care, and sorrow"—a spiritual state of rest and peace (Book of Mormon, Alma 40:12).

To LDS, family is of paramount importance both in this life and in the world to come. As a result, one of the most comforting LDS doctrines is that relationships with loving family and friends continue in the spirit world and in the resurrection. LDS find great comfort in believing that death can be sweet in that it offers relief from earthly pains and problems, joyful reunion with family and friends, and the expectation of a glorious resurrection and eternal bliss. Thus, death is merely the gateway to eternal life.

Quick and Condensed Definitions of Terms

Elders—Men holding the higher (or Melchizedek) priesthood who function as spiritual leaders.

Home teachers—Two elders who will visit monthly LDS members' homes to provide spiritual support and temporal support.

Mormon—Nickname for LDS, which relates to LDS' belief in *The Book of Mormon* (named after one of the prophets who wrote the record); while not improper to refer to them as Mormons, members of the Church prefer being called LDS.

Relief Society—Adult women of the Church, who meet monthly for gospel instruction and social and humanitarian activities.

Visiting teachers—Two members of Relief Society who contact monthly women in the ward to offer care.

Word of Wisdom—Health code (see "Views on Health and Well-Being").

Prayer

Through prayer, we not only worship God, acknowledge His goodness and power, but also petition Him to bless us according to His will and in the manner that is best for us. "The prayer of faith shall save the sick" (James 5:15). LDS believe strongly that prayer plays a significant role in both comforting and healing the sick. Members of the Church are counseled to personally pray for those who are sick and afflicted. Likewise, those who are sick are urged to exercise their own faith in prayer for healing. Congregational prayers often make mention of those who are sick and in need of special blessings. We believe that prayer is vocalized faith, and faith precedes miracles. However, it is understood that God answers all prayers according to His own purposes. Therefore, LDS believe that prayers for healing should also be expressions of faith in and acceptance of God's will for the afflicted individual.

There is a formal prayer for the sick and afflicted offered in every LDS temple. Names of those who need special blessings of healing and strength are included on a prayer roll and remembered in a special prayer offered as part of the sacred ordinances performed in these holy temples. Any person may add their own name or the name of a loved one to that prayer roll. That may be done in person at the temple or by calling the LDS temple in the area and requesting that the name be added to the prayer roll. This practice unites the faith of the believers in calling upon God to bless those in need.

In conjunction with prayer, LDS often participate in fasting, a voluntary abstinence from food, as an expression of faith. Fasting is viewed as a source of spiritual strength and a way to enhance faith and prayer. Church members are encouraged to participate in a group fast with the members of their congregation once a month, often fasting together for a specific cause or for a member of the congregation who may be in some need. Individuals may also choose to hold a personal fast to receive spiritual help. Though there is no requirement to fast, there are many patients who wish to fast but have medical conditions that prevent it. In such cases, there are often ways that they can adjust their fast to fit the situation (e.g., skipping only one meal or only eating a little).

Religious Calendar

There are no specific rituals or rites associated with any particular holy day. Worship services are held every Sunday. As Christians, Christmas and Easter are particularly significant.

Health-Promoting Practices

LDS do not use tobacco in any form, drink alcohol, tea, or coffee, or use harmful, habit-forming drugs (except under the direction of a physician for a prescribed medical treatment). There are no official prohibitions of food, such as meat. Each individual member, however, may have personal or cultural preferences. For example, a faithful LDS may choose a specific lifestyle, such as to be vegetarian or to avoid sugar or white flour or other products, but such practices are personal choices, not mandated or officially sanctioned by the Church (see "Views on Health and Well-Being").

Healing Rituals

LDS subscribe to the Bible's (James 5:14) admonition for the blessing of the sick. Elders may be called to "administer" (a common LDS term) to one who is sick. This act of "administering" to the sick person is a separate ritual or ordinance from typical prayers for or with the sick person. It is done, if possible, by two priesthood "elders" anointing the head of the sick person with consecrated olive oil and offering a prayer of faith and a pronouncement of a healing blessing upon the afflicted individual.

Other Unique Religious Beliefs, Rites, and Practices Related to Health or Illness

None.

Unique Religious Beliefs, Rites, and Practices Related to Birthing

There are no specific health or hygiene requirements or religious rituals associated with the actual birth of a child. Many, however, view child-birthing as a spiritual experience. Most LDS will, within the first few months after the birth, have the baby receive a formal "blessing" by the father and/or other priesthood holders in a worship service. This "blessing" is a prayer to God for blessings of health, strength, fulfillment of spiritual promise, and happiness in life for the child. It is not a required sacrament or ordinance of salvation. It is not uncommon for LDS parents of a baby that may die shortly after birth to request that they be able to bless and name the child, prior to (or at times shortly after) the baby's death.

Unique Religious Beliefs, Rites, or Practices Related to Childrearing

LDS believe that little children are sinless, innocent, and (as the scriptures say) "alive in Christ." As such, they have no need for baptism until they are older, have been taught religious principles, and are accountable for their own choices.

Although there is additional help and support from Church programs and activities, parents are the primary teachers for their children. To assist families in this duty, the Church encourages every family to hold a weekly family home evening where religious teachings are discussed, and bonds of family affection are strengthened. Also, families are to hold daily family prayer and scripture reading.

Unique Beliefs, Practices, and Rituals Surrounding Dying, Death, and Bereavement

The Church does not believe in euthanasia and declares that those who participate in deliberately putting to death a person who is suffering from an incurable condition or disease or by assisting someone to commit suicide violates the commandments of God. LDS, however, recognize that when dying becomes inevitable, it should be seen as a blessing and a purposeful part of eternal existence. Therefore, they should not feel obligated to extend mortal life by means that are unreasonable. These judgments are best made by family members after receiving wise and competent medical advice and seeking divine guidance through fasting and prayer.

The Church does not counsel its members against organ or tissue donation after death. That is a matter for the loved ones of the deceased to decide after receiving counsel from competent medical professionals and after receiving spiritual guidance through prayer.

The Church has no proscribed rituals or ordinances for burying and mourning the dead. Funerals or memorial services are conducted by the presiding LDS leader in consultation with the family. Such services not only reverently and joyfully memorialize the deceased but also testify, through sermons and songs of worship, of the "hope of a glorious resurrection" through Jesus Christ's redemptive love. Faithful LDS who have received sacred ordinances in LDS temples during their lifetime are generally clothed in ceremonial temple clothing for burial or cremation. Instructions and guidelines for the dressing of the deceased for burial are given to leaders of LDS congregations and done by family members, friends within the congregation, or others designated by the presiding leader of the congregation.

Role of Religious Community (Persons or Organizations) During Health Challenges

Every local LDS congregation (generally referred to as a "ward") meets weekly on Sundays for worship services. In a 3-hour block, there are three meetings that members and visitors may attend. The most important of these is what is known as Sacrament meeting. In this worship service, songs of praise are sung by the congregation, and the sacrament of the Lord's Supper is administered for the congregation. As there are no professional clergy in the LDS tradition, different members of the congregation are assigned each week to give the sermons and to offer prayers. Likewise, in the other meetings, which include gospel study classes for adults, youth, and children, members of the congregation take the responsibility to lead, teach, and minister to one another. Additionally, weekly social activities are provided for the youth, and each month the women of the congregation (Relief Society) meet for an evening of social, cultural, instructional, or service activities.

Every baptized LDS member takes upon them the solemn covenant to "bear one another's burdens, that they may be light," "mourn with those that mourn," and "comfort those that stand in need of comfort" (Book of Mormon, Mosiah 18:8–9). Therefore, it is not uncommon for members of the congregation to visit the sick, bring meals to the family, and support them in appropriate ways.

In addition to this informal and individual ministry to the sick, there are formal programs within the Church that facilitate this compassionate service. Every member (or household) is assigned "home teachers"—two lay priesthood leaders who have the responsibility to visit each month, share a spiritual message, and assist in meeting spiritual and/or temporal needs. Likewise, every adult female member of the Church is contacted monthly by "visiting teachers," two women from the Relief Society with the responsibility of supporting her. These home teachers and visiting teachers are often the "first line of defense" in knowing the needs of Church members, visiting the sick, and caring for those with special needs.

Role of Clergy During Health Challenges

Each local congregation of LDS ("ward") is presided over by a lay leader known as a bishop. A collection of several congregations or wards is known as a "stake" and is presided over by a stake president. These leaders and those who are called to assist them as counselors have the responsibility to care for the spiritual and temporal needs of the members under their jurisdiction. Therefore, they will often visit the sick members of their congregations who are in hospitals, assisted-living facilities, hospice, or other treatment centers. They go to strengthen, encourage, comfort, and pray with the sick. Also, they look for ways to help the family members of the sick. In some cases, if a member of a congregation is being treated in an area outside of the boundaries of their ward, the bishop may contact leaders of the Church in the area where treatment is being given to visit the patient and provide emotional and spiritual support.

Those who are homebound or hospitalized due to illness and unable to attend worship services may receive the ordinance of the Lord's Supper under the direction of the local ecclesiastical leader. Health care professionals can support a LDS patient's desire for this by working with that local leader (e.g., Bishop) or the patient's home teachers to make necessary arrangements. In some settings where there may be several LDS patients in the same facility, a separate worship service may be conducted by assignment of the local, presiding Church leader.

Unique Religious Aspects of Family Involvement

None.

Nursing Implications Unique to This Religious Tradition

- Health care workers who minister to LDS patients may ask them (the patient or family members) if their home or visiting teachers have been notified of their illness or hospitalization and if they would like the nurse to contact them. Sometimes, LDS patients may not be aware of their home or visiting teachers, particularly those members who are not particularly active in their congregation. They may not have been involved much with the local congregation but feel the need for spiritual support from the LDS community. In that case, the bishop of the congregation could be contacted. Addresses and phone numbers of local congregations can be found in the phonebook or at lds.org. Full-time missionaries of the Church can always be contacted to visit the sick, pray with them, and to find out the name of the leader of the patient's congregation. They can assist health care professionals in making sure that LDS patients receive appropriate fellowship and support.

- Many LDS wear special undergarments referred to as "temple garments." These are viewed as a symbolic reminder of sacred covenants made by LDS in the temple. Because of what the garments represent, patients may choose to wear them under their hospital gowns. Health care providers should be sensitive to the sacred nature of the garments by handling them in a respectful way, and when feasible, allow patients to wear them.

FOR MORE INFORMATION

Visit the Church's official websites www.mormon.org and www.lds.org.

An Introduction to the Church of Jesus Christ of LDS [DVD]. Available at http://store. lds.org/webapp/wcs/stores/servlet/Product3_715839595_10557_21084_-1 __197093

Ballard, M. R. (1993). *Our search for happiness*. Salt Lake City, UT: Deseret Book.

Ludlow, D. H. (Ed.). (1992). *Encyclopedia of Mormonism*. New York, NY: Macmillan. Available at http://eom.byu.edu/

Millet, R. L. (2007). *The vision of Mormonism: Pressing the boundaries of Christianity*. St. Paul, MN: Paragon House.

Millet, R. L., Skinner, A. C., Olson, C. F., & Top, B. L. (2011). *LDS beliefs: A doctrinal reference*. Salt Lake City, UT: Deseret Book.

19 Lutherans

CONTRIBUTOR: *The Reverend John Luoma, PhD*

NURSE REVIEWER: *Jacqueline Mickley, PhD, RN*

Theology and Social History

Lutherans are Christians whose name reflects that of Martin Luther (1483–1546), a Catholic monk who sought to reform the church using the teachings of Scripture as the primary norm for faith and life. The governing teachings of the Lutheran Church are found in the Book of Concord (1580), which contains, among other things, the Augsburg Confessions, the Small and Large Catechism, and the Apostolic, Nicene, and Athanasian creeds (historic summaries of the Christian faith). The major tenet of the Lutheran faith is that we are saved by grace through faith in Jesus Christ and not by our works. Lutherans have a distinctive way of reading the Scriptures, based on Luther's insight that God's word comes to us in two forms—law and gospel. The law as command tells people what they should do. The gospel as promise tells us what God in Christ has already done for us. Many would call the Lutheran Church "reformed Catholic" given that it sees itself as beginning a reform of the Catholic Church and continues to seek reconciliation with it.

There are over 68 million Lutherans around the world. Over the years, several different Lutheran church bodies have been established. The Evangelical Lutheran Church in America (ELCA) is the largest Lutheran group in North America with 4.5 million members; The Lutheran Church Missouri Synod has 2.3 million members.

Deity/God or Ultimate Other

Lutherans believe in the one Triune God as defined in the historic creeds: Father, Son, and Holy Spirit. God, the Father, created and loves all. God's Son, Jesus Christ, transforms lives because of his death on the cross and resurrection. God's Holy Spirit sanctifies us (the process in which God makes us his own and perfects us).

Views on Health and Well-Being

God creates us as whole persons, a unity of body, mind, and spirit. Many factors influence health such as physical and social factors, personal actions, and access to care. Worship stands at the center of the ministry of healing. God heals us as we receive God's power through the preaching of God's Word and the receiving of God's sacraments. Healing and health also come through prayer, the laying on of hands and anointing with oil, and the consolation of fellow believers. "The Church promotes health and healing and provides health care services through its social ministry organizations and congregation-based programs" (ELCA *Social Statement on Health and Healthcare*). Lutherans support disease prevention and health promotion on local, national, and international levels.

Explanations for Disease and Illness

All humans are naturally subject to disease, injury, and death. Illness and disease are the result of the human condition, personal sin, and being part of a sinful world. We are often not good stewards of our health; this negatively impacts our well-being, as well as our relationship with God, the world, and our neighbors.

The Nature of Suffering and How to Address It

Suffering is inevitable. Suffering can be due to physical problems or due to disrupted relationships with others or with God. Suffering, as viewed by Luther, is both personal and social and tied to the redemption of the world through the death of Christ. Although suffering may bring us closer to God, it can also cause some to feel separated from God. We participate in Jesus' love for humanity by "giving ourselves to others and sharing their suffering" (ELCA). To do that, we are to be compassionate to our neighbor in need of healing.

Death, Dying, and Afterlife

Death is natural and sometimes frightening. Jesus has removed the "sting" of death (1 Corinthians 15:56) through his resurrection. Lutherans believe that life with God persists even after death. "Resurrection of the dead and life everlasting" is stated in the Creeds, although an exact description of what this life is like is not possible. Anxiety about life after death is not necessary, but focus should be on God's grace and living our present life in love of God and service to others.

Care of the dying should attend to the physical, mental, and spiritual dimensions of the person. "When death is imminent, peaceful dying should become a goal of health care, sought as confidently and competently as other goals of health care through adequate palliative care and services such as hospice" (ELCA). There is no special postmortem care recommended.

Quick and Condensed Definitions of Terms

Grace—The keystone of the 16th century Reformation, based on the Bible verse, Ephesians 2:8: "For by grace you have been saved through faith, and this is not your own doing; it is the gift of God."

Sacrament—The physical sign of an unseen promise. Sacraments are rites of the church that convey God's forgiveness, life, and salvation through words and physical means. Lutherans celebrate the sacraments of Baptism and Holy Communion.

Salvation—"To be saved . . . is nothing else than to be delivered from sin, death, and the devil and to enter into the kingdom of Christ and live with him forever" (Book of Concord).

Theology of the cross—A term coined by Luther that asserts that the cross is the primary source of our knowledge of who God is and how God saves.

Real Presence—The body and blood of Christ are believed to be "truly and substantially present, in with and under" the consecrated bread and wine of Holy Communion (Augsburg Confession, Article 10).

Prayer

Prayer is an intentional way of deepening our relationship with God through various means such as quiet reflection, reciting the Scripture, or talking to Jesus, to name a few. In prayer, we are invited to ask anything and to always pray "thy will be done on earth as it is in heaven" (Matthew 6:10). God commands us to pray and promises to answer. Luther was tremendously committed to personal prayer and described his method for prayer in *A Simple Way to Pray*. Luther greatly encouraged the prayer of faith as described in James 5:13–18. Prayer may be individual or done as a group.

Religious Calendar

Christmas (Jesus' birth) and Easter (Jesus' resurrection from the dead) are important celebrations. In addition, Ash Wednesday (46 days before Easter) and Holy Week (the week leading up to Easter) are particularly important times for prayer and reflection. Lutherans observe liturgical festivals and designate days for commemoration of saints, but these are not obligatory. St. Luke Sunday is often regarded as the most significant day to talk about the ministry of healing.

Health-Promoting Practices

Lutherans vary in their adherence to health-promoting behaviors. In general, they advocate healthy living (e.g., diet, exercise) as being part of stewardship for God's creation. They observe an injunction against drunkenness (e.g., Ephesians 5:18).

Healing Rituals

Anointing with oil (James 5:14) and laying on of hands with prayer are fairly common practices for Lutherans seeking healing. Lutherans believe in the possibility of miraculous healing by God, but this is not an indication of one's faith or ability to pray. *The Evangelical Lutheran Worship, Pastoral Care* (2008) contains excellent rituals and prayers for healing (e.g., a brief order for healing, comforting the bereaved, readings, and prayers regarding healing) that a nurse could use.

Other Unique Religious Beliefs, Rites, and Practices Related to Health or Illness

None.

Unique Religious Beliefs, Rites, and Practices Related to Birthing

Contraception is generally acceptable. Lutherans have a strong pro-life stance; abortion is condoned only in very specific circumstances; adoption is encouraged. Many Lutherans practice circumcision for newborn boys but not for any specifically religious reason.

Unique Religious Beliefs, Rites, or Practices Related to Childrearing

Lutherans will baptize critically ill infants but encourage a reaffirmation of baptism at church if the child recovers. "If the possibility of life exists in a stillborn, baptism would be appropriate" (Marty, 1986, p. 143). Lutherans encourage training for early Communion and catechetical training culminating in Confirmation. They also encourage religious training at Sunday School (classes before Sunday worship) and high school youth group activities, especially mission trips where youth partner with community groups to aid the poor.

Unique Beliefs, Practices, and Rituals Surrounding Dying, Death, and Bereavement

Organ transplantation is encouraged under certain circumstances. Although a minority of Lutherans practice cremation, it is becoming increasingly acceptable. A service of Commendation for the Dying at the end of life (a service of prayer that the pastor performs just prior to death) and a service of comforting the bereaved (a prayer service any Christian might perform at gatherings prior to the funeral) are encouraged. Usually, a funeral is conducted in church by a pastor after a death, although sometimes, a memorial service is held rather than a funeral. If so, a memorial service at church is encouraged rather than at a funeral home. Such a service normally concludes at the graveside.

Role of Religious Community (Persons or Organizations) During Health Challenges

The Lutheran Church believes that the means of grace (Word and Sacrament) are the primary means of empowerment and healing.

Therefore, regular worship is encouraged. Many congregations have "prayer chains" through which they encourage the congregation to pray for the sick, as well as prayer groups that meet regularly to pray for the sick and suffering. Groups such as The Order of St. Luke (an ecumenical healing order composed of laity and clergy) and Stephen Ministry (a ministry training organization for laity) are common in Lutheran congregations. Both of these organizations provide specific study and training. Many congregations hold health fairs and provide periodic health screening and health education, often with parish nurse supervision.

Role of Clergy During Health Challenges

The Lutheran church has a strong tradition of pastoral care for the sick through clergy (typically called Pastor) or chaplains. Visitation by clergy in hospitals, nursing homes, hospices, and homes are expected. Communion may be brought to the sick wherever they reside, at home or in nursing homes, for example.

Unique Religious Aspects of Family Involvement

Martin Luther believed that the family was one of the primary structures of creation, and the church needed to do all it could to support it. He saw parents as "bishops" in their own homes and responsible for the spiritual care of their children. He developed the *Small Catechism* as a tool for the parents to teach the faith to their children. This book still provides a basic structure for Lutheran parents as they give religious training.

Nursing Implications Unique to This Religious Tradition

- The Parish Nurse movement originated in the Lutheran tradition in 1984. Its founder was Dr. Granger Westberg, a Lutheran clergyman. Every year, the annual Granger Westberg Parish Nurse Symposium provides opportunities for the continuing education of clergy, nurses, and other health care professionals. The International Parish Nurse Resource Center has excellent resources on how to approach nursing from a faith perspective (visit www.parishnurses.org.).

- Bible reading is very important. If a nurse is asked to read from the Bible, the Book of Psalms (especially Psalm 23 or 27), Gospel books (especially Luke's many stories of healing by Jesus), or Paul's letters (Romans 8 or Ephesians 1) are comforting passages to Lutherans.

- Prayer is also very important. If they are comfortable doing so, nurses may ask if the patient or family would like prayer. If a patient feels that he or she is not "good enough" or not praying "well enough" to be healed, this may indicate a spiritual crisis that needs clergy attention.

- Hymn singing is often important to Lutherans (Bach and Luther are favorite composers). Recordings could be very comforting to Lutherans, especially the elderly.

- Lutherans usually accept the ministration of any Christian clergy but may prefer a Lutheran pastor.

- Most Lutherans are buried rather than cremated, so the usual nursing care of the body after death is appropriate. Asking a close family member to assist in this care if they would like is also appropriate.

- Always ask before contacting the patient's church or a local church.

FOR MORE INFORMATION

Visit Evangelical Lutheran Church in America website at www.elca.org; note the *Social Statement on Health and Healthcare*.

Evangelical Lutheran worship, pastoral care. (2008). Minneapolis, MN: Augsburg Fortress.

Marty, M. (1983). *Health and medicine in the Lutheran tradition*. New York, NY: Crossroad.

20 **Methodists (Wesleyans)**

CONTRIBUTOR: *The Reverend Brenda Simonds, MDiv, BCC*

NURSE REVIEWER: *Sharon T. Hinton, RN, MSN*

Theology and Social History

Methodism is the theological basis for a number of Protestant Christian denominations representing about 70 million people worldwide. The United Methodist Church is the largest of these denominations. Other denominations spawned by Methodism include those within the Pentecostal and Holiness family (e.g., Nazarene churches, Salvation Army) of religions, as well as the African Methodist Episcopal Church and Wesleyan Churches. Methodism began as a movement in the 1700s in England by students at Oxford University. It was originally called "The Holy Club," where its members committed to attend their own church regularly (they were from a variety of groups, but most were from the Church of England), pray and read their Bibles daily, do a good deed for others daily, and attend their Holy Club weekly. John Wesley (1745–1791), an Anglican priest, became the organizer and leader in this movement. Wesley did not intend to create a separate church but to encourage all Christians to grow spiritually and make Christianity practical by responding to the social needs of the community. As part of their Christian commitment, The Holy Club members visited prisoners, attended to the sick, provided education to children and adults, and aided the poor. Many Anglican clergy became Methodist Anglicans in the middle 18th century. However, Methodism did not establish as a denomination in England until after John Wesley's death.

While the Methodist tradition has no exclusively Methodist doctrines, its emphasis on personal piety and practical theology are distinct characteristics of this movement. The practical emphasis requires that the Christian message be taken to where the people are and expressed by meeting the practical needs of the community. For example, Wesley went out into the mining camps in England to preach. When he arrived there, he discovered that the people suffered from illness and a lack of education. He believed that providing education to the children and health care to the workers was as important as preaching the Christian message. Wesley compiled the medical knowledge of the time period into a book entitled *Primitive Physic: An Easy and Natural Method of Curing Most Diseases*. This text was distributed by circuit riders as they visited communities to preach. This emphasis fit well in the pioneer atmosphere of the American colonies in the late 1760s when Methodist missionaries brought Methodism to America. Methodist missionaries have spread their Christian message and established churches, universities, schools, orphanages, soup kitchens, and health care facilities throughout the world.

The Bible is the primary source and norm for Christian belief within the Methodist tradition. However, it is to be interpreted in the light of tradition, personal experience, and confirmed by reason. Understanding of the meaning of the Bible and one's relationship with God develops and grows through participation in the faith community, the discipline of spiritual practices, and the implementation of the principles and ethics of the Methodist Book of Discipline. These guide the Methodist's response and obligation to people, both in the shared community and in the larger world. Methodists understand spiritual growth and transformation as an "inward holiness," which leads to an external response, which is an "outward holiness."

Deity/God or Ultimate Other

A personal relationship with God is emphasized in the Methodist tradition. It is understood that both God and humans are responsive in the relationship. Rather than being predestined, Methodists understand that they have been given free will to choose a relationship with God or not. God is responsive to our choices. God's acceptance and willingness to be personally involved with human beings is understood as a grace that is offered to everyone.

Methodists believe in one God who has many attributes that are so far beyond human understanding that they are considered mysterious. However, a trademark of Methodists' understanding of God's character is love and grace. An expression of God's love and grace is seen both in Jesus Christ (who represents God's willingness to become human to demonstrate God's love for humanity) and in the Holy Spirit (which is God's spirit that dwells within humans and gives them comfort and guidance throughout life). A goal of the human journey is to strive for complete holiness or perfection—sanctification. It is generally understood that this perfection is a goal and rarely obtainable in this life, yet God's prevenient grace is offered to us in our imperfection.

Methodists understand communication with God in multiple ways. Primarily, they use prayer. Methodists also communicate with God and understand God through music, sacraments, rituals, nature, relationships, and acts of service.

Views on Health and Well-Being

A Methodist's view of health and well-being is holistic. "Wesley often preached about the restoration of the soul through inward and outward health." (United Methodist Committee on Relief [UMCOR]-Health, 2009, p. 3). Methodists understand that the role of religion is to promote both spiritual well-being and physical health. Health is promoted with a combination of spiritual practices, discipline, and devotion, alongside preventative and restorative health care. Congregations are encouraged to develop health ministries to serve members of the congregations as well as people in the surrounding community.

Explanations for Disease and Illness

Methodists believe that illness and disease are a result of living in a broken world. Methodists do not adhere to the belief that God punishes by giving us illnesses and disease. However, Methodists do believe in evil. They understand that from free will, humans do not always choose a path that promotes health or positive relationships with God and others. There are consequences to our choices both historically and currently. Natural catastrophes or unexplainable illness are attributable to evil. Methodist theology does not suggest that God gives people illness as a result of their bad choice(s) or for their sinful nature. Instead, God is with us in our illness bringing comfort, care, and healing.

The Nature of Suffering and How to Address It

Suffering is defined by the individual. Suffering can be physical, emotional, spiritual, or a combination. According to a Methodist perspective, suffering is meant to be alleviated out of Christian compassion. It would not be expected of a person to endure suffering for the sake of being a good Christian. However, there are certainly opportunities for spiritual growth in and through suffering. Suffering can challenge our theology and our perspective allowing us to rethink our beliefs and recommit to new and deeper understanding. Suffering can also challenge our understanding of a benevolent God and cause us spiritual distress especially if care and relief is not given to us by compassionate caregivers. Methodist doctrine encourages congregational support of suffering individuals as members of the body of Christ.

Death, Dying, and Afterlife

Death is seen as the enemy. Life is precious and is to be preserved. However, when life cannot be preserved, hope is found in anticipating that there is life after death. There is no standard picture of what life after death will be like except that it is understood to be free of pain and suffering. God promises to be with us "through the valley of death" and bring comfort in our sorrow.

Quick and Condensed Definitions of Terms

Methodist terminology reflects Protestant Christian language use.

Prayer

Prayer is a form of direct communication with God. Prayer is both personal and corporate. Prayer is often spontaneous, but formalized common prayers are often used in community worship services. *The Lord's Prayer* is a common prayer used in the Methodist tradition. Prayer is also used for purposes of confession or repentance, petition, praise, and thanksgiving. In formal settings, prayers of confession are always followed by words of forgiveness and assurance.

Prayers for healing and health are part of Methodist tradition. In worship services, prayer requests are solicited, and prayers of petition are made on behalf of individuals and groups. Prayer requests are listed in congregational newsletters and often prayed for by a prayer chain of church members.

Religious Calendar

The most holy time on the Christian liturgical calendar is the Lenten Season, which starts with Ash Wednesday and ends with the celebration on Easter Sunday. Ash Wednesday is a time of repentance, and observers usually attend a service where they receive ashes on their forehead to symbolize their repentance for sins and shortcomings. The Lenten Season is a time when Christians reflect on their relationship with God. It is a time to reflect on priorities and renew commitment to God and the Christian principles that guide lifestyle, values, and priorities.

Christmas is celebrated with special music, pageants, and services. It is a season when Christians are reminded of God's love, which is symbolized by the gathering of family and friends to honor relationships. Families and individual faith communities establish multiple traditions to celebrate Christmas.

Health-Promoting Practices

Methodists understand the body as a "temple of God." Their theology understands the connection between body and spirit. Methodists are encouraged by their faith community to seek health care. Practices of moderation are promoted. Although Methodists are encouraged to restrain from unhealthy eating habits, smoking, excessive alcohol, and drug abuse, these vices would not be labeled as sin. From the beginning of the Methodist movement, Methodists have tended to be passionate about preventative medicine, encouraging healthy lifestyles and exercise. The denomination promotes health in congregations through faith community nursing, health advocates, and programs to improve the physical, mental, spiritual, financial, and social health of members of the congregation and the surrounding community.

Healing Rituals

Healing services are common within the Methodist tradition. During the service, a pastor, faith community nurse, or health advocate may say a prayer for healing and place oil on the forehead of the one for whom prayer is offered. However, a Methodist would most likely welcome prayers for healing from anyone who would be comfortable offering a prayer on their behalf. Because the anointing of oil in the Methodist tradition is not a sacrament, anyone who is comfortable could also honor the patients by blessing them with oil and prayer. The oil is a symbol of God's healing touch and reminds us of God's ability to heal. Formal healing services are also offered in Methodist congregations.

Familiar passages from the Bible can bring comfort and function as part of a healing prayer ritual. Therefore, patients would often like access to a Bible or Christian literature. They would often welcome being read to from the Bible.

Other Unique Religious Beliefs, Rites, and Practices Related to Health or Illness

Within the Methodist faith tradition are people of different cultures and nationalities. Methodists are pluralistic and affirming of honoring people's cultural heritage. Therefore, Methodist congregations may adopt cultural practices that have special meaning that are unique to the culture of the community the church serves.

Unique Religious Beliefs, Rites, and Practices Related to Birthing

Methodists practice infant baptism. The baptism is intended to be done in the congregation where the community participates and embraces the baby as a member of the community in which the baby will receive care, nurture, and education. If a baby is ill or terminal, however, it would be important for the Methodist parents to have their baby baptized as a symbol of God's love and acceptance for the baby. Methodists do not, however, believe that their baby will not go to heaven if they are not baptized. Given that only clergy perform baptisms, a referral to a chaplain should be made at such time if possible.

Methodists are not united on their beliefs about abortion. However, the *United Methodist Book of Discipline* affirms the sanctity of life while honoring a woman's right to decide for herself regarding abortion. The *Discipline* requires that the woman receive support and consultation as she makes this difficult decision. The *Discipline* forbids abortion to be used as a way of gender selection or birth control.

Unique Religious Beliefs, Rites, or Practices Related to Childrearing

None.

Unique Beliefs, Practices, and Rituals Surrounding Dying, Death, and Bereavement

Visitation of the sick and dying is an important part of Methodist tradition. Funeral or memorial services are part of the bereavement ritual.

There are no requirements from the Methodist religion regarding the type or form of burial or disposition of the body. Likewise, there are no religious requirements for or against organ and tissue donation. These are a matter of personal choice and so honored by the Methodist community.

Role of Religious Community (Persons or Organizations) During Health Challenges

Methodists meet regularly as a congregation at least each Sunday for worship in a church building. The service consists of music, prayer, readings from the Bible, a sermon, and periodically, they observe communion or the Lord's Supper.

Some congregations have Faith Community Nurses as staff members who are registered nurses with active licensure and additional training focusing on working in a congregational setting. Faith community nurses may or may not be members of the congregation or denomination in which they serve. In congregations without faith community nurses, health advocates (nonregistered nurses such as Licensed Vocational/ Practical Nurses, allied health, retired health care providers and others interested in specific health practices such as exercise or nutrition) may provide health ministry. They serve a unique role in the congregation, helping parishioners with health-related issues. Some congregations also have Steven's Ministers who are trained lay visitors who visit the sick.

Role of Clergy During Health Challenges

Usually, Methodist clergy visit members of their congregations in the hospital. Faith Community Nurses often provide additional visitation and support.

Unique Religious Aspects of Family Involvement

The role of family members during times of illness is more determined by culture than by the Methodist beliefs.

Nursing Implications Unique to This Religious Tradition

- Familiar Scriptures that remind believers of God's love, acceptance, and presence with us through difficult times would generally be welcomed. It would be an affirmation of one's faith when fear and doubt might be felt. Particularly comforting Bible passages include Psalms and the Lord's Prayer (Matthew 6:9–13).

- Prayer (and even an anointing with oil) can be offered by a nurse who shares with the patient a belief in the efficacy of these rituals (see "Healing Rituals" for more information about the symbolism and practice of anointing).

- Some Methodists may welcome receiving the communion at the bedside. The nursing staff can inform the Methodist pastor or chaplain regarding the patient's ability to take food by mouth, as the ritual includes a small piece of bread and a small amount of grape juice. On Ash Wednesdays, Methodist patients will most often value receiving ashes by a pastor or chaplain even if they are unable to attend a service.

- Given the cultural plurality of Methodists, it is important to ask each Methodist patient and or their family about rituals and practices that are meaningful to them and try to accommodate them.

- Faith community nurses and congregational health ministries are a valuable resource for providing spiritual support, health education, augmentation of discharge planning, and community resource and referral information.

FOR MORE INFORMATION

Visit the United Methodist Church (UMC) website at http://www.umc.org and the UMC health ministry website at http://www.gbgm-umc.org/parishnursing

The book of discipline of the United Methodist Church. (2008). Nashville, TN: United Methodist Publishing House.

Madden, D. (2008). *'Inward and outward health': John Wesley's holistic concept of medical science, the environment, and holy living.* London: Epworth Press.

Marquardt, M. (1992). *John Wesley's social ethics.* Nashville, TN: Abingdon Press.

Stokes, M. B. (1989). *Major United Methodist beliefs.* Nashville, TN: Abingdon Press.

UMCOR-Health. (2009). *Introduction to health ministry for United Methodist congregations.* New York, NY: UMCOR.

21   Modern Pagans*

CONTRIBUTOR: *Carol T. Kirk, RN, BSN, MS, CLNC*

Theology and Social History

Paganism or Neo-Paganism refers to a grouping of disparate religions that share some common attributes. In general, Pagan religions (1) are polytheistic, (2) view the material world as a manifestation of the Divine, and (3) honor the Divine Feminine. Most forms of Paganism are highly experiential in nature; that is, what is important is the individual's direct experiences with the Divine and the Cosmos. Pagan traditions lack a set dogma or set of holy scriptures.

Modern Paganism has its roots in the esoteric movements in Western Europe during the 18th and 19th centuries. However, it was largely unknown outside of very small groups of individuals until the repeal of the anti-Witchcraft laws in Britain in 1951. During the 1960s and 1970s, the Pagan movement reached across the Atlantic to the United States and Canada as well as to Australia and New Zealand where it found support within both the Feminist movement and the growth of ecological consciousness. Within paganism, there are successes in reconstructing historical *polytheistic* religions in the modern world, such as the Kemetic (Egyptian), Hellenismos (Greek), Nova Roma (Roman), and Celtic traditions.

It is now estimated that there are between 1 and 2 million individuals worldwide who self-identify as being Pagan with over 300,000 of those being in the United States. Recent surveys indicate that modern Paganism is one of the fastest growing religious movements in the world. Studies of the demographics of the various Pagan religions have indicated that the majority of practitioners are middle class and college educated. Although Paganism has tended to attract a younger group of followers, there are also those across the age range who have found the spirituality they are seeking in Pagan practices. Families are now raising children within Pagan faiths, so it is not unusual to find multigenerational Pagan families.

Modern Pagans have faced significant challenges in their freedom to practice their religion largely due to misunderstandings about the nature of Paganism. Practitioners of Wicca and modern religious Witchcraft have been targeted for religious discrimination because of the misapprehension that these groups engage in human sacrifice and other diabolical practices. As a result, Pagans may be reluctant to admit to their spiritual beliefs or wear religious symbols openly for fear of persecution. This can make it difficult for Pagans to find others in their area who share their beliefs and thus a sense of isolation is felt by Pagans in a non-Pagan community, which often views Paganism with hostility.

Deity/God or Ultimate Other

Modern Paganism is largely theistic in nature, although it would be incorrect to say that all Pagans are theistic. The majority of Pagans are either duotheistic (such as the Wiccan worship of the God and Goddess) or they are polytheistic, choosing to worship Deities drawn from the many different classical pantheons. Some might choose to limit their worship to a single pantheon such as the Kemetic worship of the Gods of ancient Egypt. Others might develop relationships with Deities from various pantheons to which they feel drawn. However, there are also those who view the Deities as Jungian archetypes rather than as actual Divine beings.

Pagans believe that they are capable of having direct knowledge and intercourse with their Gods because those Gods are immanent or present here in the material world. A Pagan does not require a minister or priest to act as a go-between for them when interacting with their Gods. Many of the Pagan religions consider each of their followers to be their own priest or priestess.

Pagans believe that the Gods need human beings, and human beings need the Gods. The relationship with Deity is intensely personal and requires a give and take between the individual and the Divine. One can connect with the Divine through prayer, through ritual, through meditation, through dreams, or in many other ways.

Views on Health and Well-Being

Most Pagans view health holistically: One must be healthy in mind and spirit as well as body to be truly well. This holistic view values meditation, yoga, Reiki, and other practices. Some Pagans view Western medicine and particularly modern pharmaceuticals with suspicion and prefer to avoid taking medications when possible if herbal remedies are available. Many of these same individuals may be taking regular herbal supplements and fail to understand the issue of drug interactions between their herbs and the medications that the physician might prescribe. It would behoove the nurse to explore any health supplements that the Pagan patient might be taking in order to ensure that no unexpected drug reactions occur. In addition, the nurse should be willing to help the Pagan patient explore possible alternatives to standard pharmaceuticals with their physician to ensure that the patient will be compliant with the agreed-upon treatment regimen.

Explanations for Disease and Illness

Pagans tend to be well-educated and pragmatic people who answer questions of causality and "why?" with answers from modern scientific knowledge. In general, Pagans do not believe that disease and illness is something visited upon them by vengeful Gods or because of their sins, nor do they view illness as something visited upon them by the Divine in order to "make them stronger." However, a small minority of Pagans may believe that they are suffering in this lifetime because of something that they did in a past life for which they are now atoning.

The Nature of Suffering and How to Address It

The majority of Pagans simply acknowledge that suffering happens, often through no action of their own. Suffering is something to be handled with dignity, inner strength, and the help of the Gods.

Death, Dying, and Afterlife

There are differing schools of thought within modern Paganism about what happens after death. Therefore, it would be important to explore with the patient exactly how they think about death and what comes after death. While a few Pagans believe that death is the end, most Pagans view death not as an end, but as a beginning. One might die and go to one of the Pagan equivalents of the concept of Heaven. For example, for the Asatru, it would be Valhalla, for a Hellenic Reconstructionist, perhaps the Elysian Fields. Many others hold to the idea of reincarnation: they are born, they die, and they are born again. Wiccans tend to believe that when they die, they go to the Summerlands where the soul can rest and consider the lessons learned in their lifetime before they are reborn into this world again. Pagans have no concept of a place of eternal torment. For most Pagans, comfort might come from being reminded that the death of the body is not the death of the spirit and a reminder that the spirit will be reunited and know those they have loved and lost can be comforting.

Quick and Condensed Definitions of Terms

Animism—The belief that souls exist; more commonly, the belief that both animate creatures and inanimate objects or concepts may themselves possess souls.

Asatru—Modern revival of Scandinavian or Germanic Paganism.

Druidry—Modern Pagan movement based loosely on what is known of the historical Druids augmented with the philosophies of the 19th century esoteric movement in Britain.

Henotheism—Worshipping a single Divinity while acknowledging that other Divinities exist. Less commonly, means worshipping multiple Divinities while perceiving one of these Divinities to be supreme over the others.

Immanent—Existing or remaining within; inherent. In theological terms, an opposite of transcendent. An immanent Divinity is present within Its creation.

Pantheism—Belief that the universe and Divinity are one and the same: that the Divine is all that is, and that all that is is, in turn, Divine.

Panentheism—This view between strict *theism* and *pantheism*. The panentheist viewpoint is that Divinity is both transcendent and immanent. That is, Divinity is seen as being present throughout the universe, whereas at the same time, the Divine encompasses more than the universe, so that it is possible to distinguish between the universe and Divinity.

Theism–Belief that Divinity actually exists and possesses the attributes of being a person (e.g., "belief in a personal God"); generally, theists believe that the universe was created by their personified Divinity and that this Divinity transcends creation. Subcategories include: monotheism (single divinity); duotheism (the two divinities may enjoy a complementary relationship, as is seen in the relationship between the God and the Goddess in Wicca, or be adversaries, as is seen in Zoroastrianism or Manichaeism); and polytheism (*"hard" polytheism*—multiple Divinities that exist are distinctly individual and separate, and *"soft" polytheism*—multiple Divinities are but aspects or manifestations of some greater Whole).

Wicca—Is a Neopagan religion and a form of modern witchcraft. Wicca is typically a duotheistic religion, worshipping a Goddess and a God, who are traditionally viewed as the Triple Goddess and Horned God.

Prayer

As a vital practice for many modern Pagans, prayer allows Pagans to have close relationships with their Deities and to ask for their help with difficult situations. Prayer is generally an individual activity. However, if the individual is a member of a group or is known in the local Pagan community, prayers may be offered by community or group members as well. Because most Pagans follow their beliefs outside of groups, it may be that they will not have visits from any of their faith group leaders; however, for those who are part of established groups, the leader(s) of that group may visit the sick. If so, it is possible that that group leader or member of the group might pray with the individual.

Religious Calendar

The observance of holy days will vary among Pagan traditions. Perhaps the best known of the Pagan observances is the so-called Wheel of the Year, which includes a total of eight holidays that fall on the following schedule in the Northern Hemisphere: Yule—December 21–23 (Winter solstice); Imbolc—February 2; Ostara—March 21–23 (Spring Equinox); Beltane— May 1; Midsummer—June 21–23 (Summer Solstice); Lammas—August 1; Mabon—September 21–23 (Fall Equinox); Samhain—October 31. For those who follow the Wheel of the Year, these are times for the group to gather together for special rituals to mark the meaning of the holiday. Individuals will mark these days with special rituals of their own. For instance, Samhain is a time to honor the ancestors and the beloved dead, and a common custom is the "Dumb Supper," when a plate is laid at the table for those ancestors or loved ones who are no longer with them. In addition, Witches and Wiccans tend to celebrate the full moon each month.

Health-Promoting Practices

Although there are no prescribed or proscribed lifestyle practices, individual Pagans may engage in a variety of health-promoting practices based on their personal understanding of their spiritual path. Some of these include vegetarianism or veganism, meditation, yoga, Reiki, and dietary supplementation.

Healing Rituals

A Pagan patient may wish to pray or perform a ritual to help restore their health. Magic, the God-given ability to act on their own to attain desired outcomes, may be what the Pagan patient wants. Magic involves the raising and shaping of energy to achieve a desired result. A Pagan patient may wish to charge a candle, engage in chanting, or some other magical act as part of their recovery.

Other Unique Religious Beliefs, Rites, and Practices Related to Health or Illness

It is possible for Pagans to engage in a ritual observance without any symbols of their faith around them. However, it might be comforting for the sick to be able to have some of the things that would normally be a part of their ritual such as soft music, perhaps some chanting, incense, candles, or even a small altar could be set up on a bedside table. If the patient desires the opportunity to engage in ritual practice during a hospital stay, it would be appropriate to ask the patient what he or she would need for the ritual, and to come to an agreement on what would be possible given hospital rules and regulations. If possible, and if the patient desires their presence, family, friends, or other members of their group could be permitted to attend as well. Then, it is a matter of giving the patient a place for privacy for the length of the ritual.

Unique Religious Beliefs, Rites, and Practices Related to Birthing

Although no religiously mandated rites or practices related to birthing exist, many Pagans prefer to have either a home birth or birth in a birthing center where the surroundings are less clinical than in a hospital. Often the mothers like soft music or chanting to welcome the infant. Some birthing centers make allowances for Pagan parents to have candles or incense in the birthing room by simply removing any oxygen containers while the flame is present. Mothers may wish to have close friends or family present for the event as well. The purpose is to return to the more natural birthing process. Given the goal of a healthy child and mother, however, appropriate intervention will not be refused if a problem occurs with the birth.

There is no Pagan stricture against abortion. This is considered to be an individual choice between the woman, her physician, and her Gods. While Pagans treasure their children, they also realize that there are times when it is better for a child not to be born. On the other hand, they also recognize that both partners in a sexual relationship have a responsibility to do their best to prevent conception if a child is not wanted.

Unique Religious Beliefs, Rites, or Practices Related to Childrearing

Although there are no religious strictures regarding childrearing in modern Pagan practice, many Pagans eschew physical correction such as spanking and prefer to guide and correct their children through less physical means. Pagan children are encouraged to explore, to be creative, and to become the person they were meant to be. Some Pagans will rear their children within the Pagan faith. Others may choose not to include the child in their spiritual practices until the child is of an age to decide. Checking with the parent as to whether their child is being raised within their faith is important.

Unique Beliefs, Practices, and Rituals Surrounding Dying, Death, and Bereavement

Because many Pagans view death as a normal part of the cycle of life, they feel that death, like birth, should be removed when possible from the clinical setting. If the patient cannot be removed from the hospital, allowing the family to be present and to share in the dying process is very important. Hospice is also a valid choice for the terminally ill Pagan. The family may wish to pray or sing with the dying patient or have some incense or light candles. Pagan family members or members of their faith group may wish to be able to wash and prepare the body after death. This should be discussed with the family.

Because many Pagans are interested in ecological issues, many Pagans opt for either cremation or for green burials. The goal of a natural or green burial is to return the body to the earth in a manner that does not inhibit decomposition and allows the body to recycle naturally. This means that no embalming will be performed, and the body will be placed in a wooden or cardboard casket that is buried directly in the earth rather than a vault. Not all states have green or natural burial sites available. There is an excellent resource on the subject with information on available green cemeteries at http://www.naturalburial.coop/. Some states permit the body to be buried on private land if certain restrictions are met. Many states permit the placement of cremated remains on private land. Check with the authorities in the appropriate state of residence for particulars.

There is no specific Pagan stricture against suicide or assisted suicide. The vast majority of Pagans would consider that suicide in the face of a temporary condition would be a terrible shame; suicide when faced with terminal illness is not. In the case of a terminally ill patient, the choice to end one's life belongs to the patient and their Gods.

Role of Religious Community (Persons or Organizations) During Health Challenges

Paganism consists of widely divergent spiritual traditions with widely divergent practices. Some groups will have monthly religious gatherings, some less frequently, some even more frequently. Many Pagans practice on their own with no group affiliation of any sort. Most Pagan groups are quite small and will meet in someone's home or at a secluded place outdoors. If the patient is a member of a coven, grove, or other Pagan group, their group leader(s) may assume this role just as would other clergy.

Role of Clergy During Health Challenges

One of the most difficult things for most Pagan patients in the hospital setting is the lack of Pagan clergy to help them address spiritual questions they might have. Few trained Pagan clergy are available at the moment, although that is changing. Furthermore, most hospitals typically do not keep a list of local Pagan clergy to contact in need.

Unique Religious Aspects of Family Involvement

Because of a history of persecution, Pagans may be reluctant to discuss their spirituality with someone who is not themselves Pagan. They may also not wish to have their family or friends know about their faith if this is a source of conflict. A difficulty for families of Pagan patients is confidentiality regarding the patient's religious choice. Disclosure of Pagan religiosity has caused families to break apart, estrangement, lost jobs, and hate crimes. Querying family and friends about a patient's faith is inappropriate, unless the patient indicates otherwise.

Nursing Implications Unique to This Religious Tradition

- Pagan patients may refrain from self-disclosure of religiosity due to fear of persecution (during spiritual assessment or other times).

- While some hospital chaplains may try to support Pagan patients, most Pagans are extremely uncomfortable working with clergy of mainstream religions. Nurses could be able to provide spiritual support when needed and requested if they identify various Pagan groups in their locality who might be willing to be on-call for Pagan patients.

- A Pagan's faith group is like a family of choice. Pagans may feel closer to those in their coven, grove, or hearth than they do to their birth family. Clinical policies should permit members of their faith group to be with them, if the patient desires.

- Most pagans will prefer to die away from a clinical setting and often desire a green burial (see "Unique Beliefs, Practices, and Rituals Surrounding Dying, Death, and Bereavement").

FOR MORE INFORMATION

Adler, M. (2006). *Drawing down the moon: Witches, druids, goddess-worshippers and other pagans in America.* New York, NY: Penguin.

Higginbotham, J., & Higginbotham, R. (2002). *Paganism: A guide to earth-centered religions.* Woodbury, MA: Llewellyn Worldwide.

Hutton, R. (2001). *Triumph of the moon: A history of modern pagan witchcraft.* New York, NY: Oxford Press.

Hutton, R. (2011). *Blood and mistletoe: A history of the Druids.* New Haven, CT: Yale University Press.

Paxson, D. L., & Bonewits, I. (2006). *Essential Astaru: Walking the path of Norse paganism.* New York, NY: Citadel Press.

NOTE

*It is not easy to summarize the beliefs and practices of modern Pagans in this limited space. Paganism includes multiple traditions with few similarities and enormous differences.

22 Muslims

CONTRIBUTOR: *Muhamad Ali, PhD*

NURSE REVIEWER: *Anna Garton, RN*

Theology and Social History

The word *Islam* means submission to God; in Arabic, it shares the same root as the word "peace." Islam is a religion and a way of life sent from God to the Prophet, Muhammad (circa 570 to June 8, 632). Although Islam originated in what is today called Saudi Arabia, it has spread to the world by ways of expansion, teaching, trade, marriage, and cultural interactions. With around 1.5 billion adherents internationally, Islam is the second largest religion and fastest growing one today. Most Muslims (adherents of Islam) live in Middle Eastern and Southern and Southeast Asian countries, as well as Sub-Saharan Africa, but Muslim communities are growing in Europe, North America, and elsewhere. Most Muslims are of the Sunni denomination, while 10%–20% are Shia, or of a smaller sector (e.g., the mystical tradition of Sufi). Although these denominations share similar practices, variations in beliefs result from variations in the *hadiths* (or reports about Mohammad) passed down by scholars and religious leaders.

Muslims believe that Islam is the completed and perfected religion that incorporates Judaism and Christianity. They believe that Muhammed was the last messenger sent by God. Islamic law, or *Shari'a*, offers Muslims not only creed, but also a way of living and guidance for society (e.g., from directives on banking to care for the environment). *Shari'a* is received from the *Qur'an* (holy book) and *Sunnah* (acts, sayings, and traditions of Muhammad and his followers). *Shari'a* identifies five "pillars of faith," acts of worship to which the Muslim is obligated. These pillars include making an oath stating that there is no other God but Allah and that the Prophet Muhammed is his messenger; praying five times a day; paying 2.5% of one's income to charity if one has some savings; making a pilgrimage to Mecca (where Islam began) at least once during one's lifetime, if possible; and fasting from sunrise to sunset during the month of Ramadan (if it is not deleterious to health). The primary objectives of Islamic law are protection of life, religion, body and mind, property, family, and lineage.

Deity/God or Ultimate Other

Islam is a monotheistic religion that believes in one God, *Allah*. (In Arabic, *Allah* means God.) God is concerned about the personal life of the individual as well as their social life. Muslims communicate with God through prayers regularly and, occasionally, according to human circumstances. God also communicates with the individual through written words as recorded in the *Qur'an* as well as through natural and social phenomena from which an individual can learn.

The *Qur'an* states that human beings are not originally sinful, but they are forgetful. Because of this forgetfulness, they need to be reminded of the omnipotent presence of God to help them through life. A Muslim is someone who submits to God and acts accordingly in goodness and patience. The *Qur'an* serves as guidance for the believer. "The Qur'an has its cure . . . ." "God loves those who repent and are clean." "Don't destroy things on earth." These are some of the *Qur'anic* passages with health implications.

Views on Health and Well-Being

Faith and health were described by Prophet Mohammad as the most important attributes one could possess. It is a duty to protect one's health; indeed, one will be punished if at the Judgment Day one is deemed to have misused health. To be healthy is to be physically, spiritually, and socially well. Health involves having the body, which is in a state of dynamic equilibrium, keep its potential. This potential is supported by eating nutritious food, maintaining physical and mental fitness, personal security, and such. Guidelines exist on what to eat and drink to maintain this equilibrium and cleanliness. These guidelines are outlined in the *Qur'an*, *Sunnah*, and *hadith*, and most Muslims will have firm views about how these relate to their daily lives. To be spiritually healthy is to practice patience, repentance, forgiving, and resilience. Health also involves making choices for good and against evil. For example, healthy eyes will focus on what is beneficial, not on forbidden objects. Health also requires balancing individual interests with societal needs; indeed, the needs of the individual and of society are deeply interrelated. Hence, for Muslims, there is a responsibility to care for their own, especially those who are marginalized by poverty, disability, and illness.

Explanations for Disease and Illness

Disease can be mainly physical, but often there can also be spiritual and mental components affecting the disease process. Mental health problems can be attributed to greed, lust, worry, confusion, uncontrolled desire, anger, arrogance, lying, enmity, fear of death. Physical illness manifests when the requirements of prayer, sleep, lifestyle, and faith become out of balance. Prophet Muhammad said, "God has not created a disease without creating a cure for it." This saying is interpreted to mean that all diseases can be cured if it is God's will. Muslims rely on prayers of supplication (dissimilar to the faith healing practiced by many Christians), as well as medical science for this cure. Because of this, Muslim physicians have contributed greatly to science over the centuries. The Prophet Muhammad, who himself was sick prior to his death at age 63, recited specific *Qur'anic* verses and made supplication or intercessory prayer on behalf of others who were sick.

The Nature of Suffering and How to Address It

Suffering occurs when one lacks the essential needs in life: food, water, housing, clothing, and so forth. Depending on circumstances, this can also include education, clean environment, social order, and political stability. All Muslims are reminded that illness is a test from God, to show them a way to devote more time and energy to the worship of God and a closer adherence to his prescribed ways. The Muslim finds solace and comfort in the awareness of pre-ordainment and that tests and trials sent by God to them in this life will impact on their ability to be admitted to *Jannah* (heaven) on the Day of Judgment. Muslims address illness and suffering first by following the religious prescriptions for healing (e.g., eating and drinking certain foods, reading *Qur'an*) alongside medical therapies. When the patient and his or her community have done all they can to resolve the problem, then they accept that *Allah* has the final say—"*in sha Allah*" (meaning "by God's will"). This is reflected in the motto of some Islamic hospitals: "We care, but *Allah* heals."

Death, Dying, and Afterlife

Muslims believe that every physical body dies. When this occurs, the spirit lies in slumber until the Day of Judgment. On the Day of Judgment, rewards and punishments according to the faith and actions during their lives are determined. Muslims believe in an afterlife that is considered beautiful and blissful (in paradise), or devastating (in hell). Muslims spend considerable time praying for admission to paradise, to join loved ones, the Prophets, and to be in the presence of God. Dying patients will be comforted by a strong belief that they will live again. Death is a path to another life, an everlasting life. For those who feel they have sins, they can pray and ask forgiveness from God. God is all-forgiving and all-merciful.

Quick and Condensed Definitions of Terms

Do'a or *Shalat*—Prayer, recited softly and sincerely in one's heart in his/her own language.

Allah—The name of the single and only true God.

Shari'a—Islamic law, do's and don'ts in this life in order to be healthy physically, spiritually, and socially.

Ka'ba—the cube-shaped sanctuary located in the city of Mecca, toward which Muslims direct their regular prayers.

Qur'an—Holy book containing verbatim in Arabic the words of God spoken to Muhammad; the most authoritative source of *Shari'a*. This text in another language is called a translation of the *Qur'an*, but is not actually a *Qur'an*.

Wudhu—Making ablution or washing with clean water the face, hands, lower arms, feet, face, mouth, nose, ears, and hair of the head (quickly); usually performed before prayers or handling the *Qur'an*.

Prayer

Prayer, or *Do'a*, is the means by which a Muslim asks God for protection, blessing, recovery, or anything they wish for in this life or in paradise. Prayers have psychological impact on a Muslim who believes in its power. As one of the five pillars of faith, a Muslim will pray five times a day: at dawn, midday, late afternoon, after sunset, and late evening while facing Mecca. These prayers are obligatory, and it is a sin to fail to pray these prayers. Prayers can be corporate or be individual, in Arabic or in the language of the believer. Prayer typically involves saying ritual prayers that glorify Allah and ask for a blessing and reciting chapters from the *Qur'an*. For those who are able, these prayers are said during varying postures (standing, bending, kneeling, prostration). For those who are unable, the prayers can be completed from a sitting or lying position. Prayers are to be said in a clean environment, after cleansing oneself observing prescribed ritual ablutions. Persons who are menstruating or physically or mentally incapable of saying the obligatory prayers are exempt from doing so. Those who are unable to do so for some temporary reason are expected to make up the missed prayers.

Religious Calendar

Ramadan, the ninth month in the lunar Islamic calendar, celebrates when Muhammad began to receive the revelations written in the *Qur'an*. Whereas *Ramadan* began on August 1 in 2011, it will begin 11 days earlier each subsequent year. During this 29–30 days, Muslims fast, seek forgiveness, practice charity, and observe religious devotional practices (e.g., reading the entire *Qur'an*) as they seek to draw closer to *Allah*.

At the close of Ramadan, the Eid al-Fitri, the Festival of Returning to the Natural State of Being, is celebrated with feasting, visiting friends and family, and gift giving—including giving food to the poor. Seventy days later, the Eid al-Adha, the Festival of Sacrifice, commemorates the willingness of Abraham to sacrifice his son. On these two festivals, Muslims pray together, listen to sermons, and have a communal meal and play for families and children.

Health-Promoting Practices

Halal, or permissible food, includes any meat (except pork, and that which contains ample amounts of blood) from an animal without claws personally hunted or slaughtered by others in the name of God. It is recommended that one eat in moderation. One is encouraged to think of the stomach as being divided into three portions, one each for food, fluid, and air, to discourage overeating. Drinking alcohol is forbidden. As smoking and illicit drugs are considered to damage health, most Muslims will refrain from these practices.

Healing Rituals

There are no specific healing rituals, but families and imams may want to recite the Qur'an in the presence of the ill person. Muslims pray for strength, hope, and patience for the sick, potentially in the presence of the sick person, who is comforted by this. They may also seek natural-based remedies prescribed by their faith (e.g., the ingestion or application of honey, dates, herbs, olives, [camel] milk, black cumin, zam zam water [sourced from the holy city of Mecca]).

Other Unique Religious Beliefs, Rites, and Practices Related to Health or Illness

Sometimes Muslims make ablution (*Wudhu*) not just before prayer or handling the *Qur'an* but also perform it anytime when needed—including when sick. *Wudhu* puts the Muslim in a state of ritual purity and can wash the distractions of this life away so as to fully communicate with Allah.

Unique Religious Beliefs, Rites, and Practices Related to Birthing

Although the fetus does not become a soul until the 120th day after conception, most Islamic scholars posit that postcoital contraception is unacceptable. Acceptable methods would include rhythm and barrier methods. In the context of a valid marriage, fertility is a duty; hence, certain fertility treatments are encouraged if needed, but using donor material for conception is disliked as it is akin to adultery.

When birthing, mothers are encouraged to recite Islamic recitations such as *bismilla* ("In the name of God, the beneficent, the merciful") and other prayers they know to ease the process. Once the baby is born, someone (father, relative, or a religious leader invited) recites a call to prayer (*adhan*) by the ears of the newly born.

Male circumcision is obligatory and may be performed at different possible times prior to age 7. Female circumcision is not described in *Qur'an* or other holy books.

Unique Religious Beliefs, Rites, or Practices Related to Childrearing

Childrearing differs from culture to culture. In general, children are taught the *Qur'an*, basic Arabic, basic Islamic beliefs and practices, and morality. Parents bring their children to mosques or Islamic schools for this education, as well as provide it in the home. Once children reach puberty, they are expected to observe the rituals of Ramadan and daily prayers. However, boys as young as 10 years may begin praying regularly. Muslims do not adopt children as it disrespects lineage. Muslims will become a caretaker for orphans, but ensure these children will keep their last name. Extended family, when possible, will care for widows and their children.

Unique Beliefs, Practices, and Rituals Surrounding Dying, Death, and Bereavement

When a Muslim is near death, the patient is encouraged to say *Shahada* (i.e., "There is no God except Allah, and Muhammed is his prophet). A *Qur'anic* passage (any passage) is read, and the dying person is encouraged to repent and anticipate *Allah's* mercy. After the death, the body is cleansed and enshrouded in three white sheets (for men) and sheets plus clothing (five layers for women). This ritual cleansing is typically done by family members of the same gender as the deceased as well as a trusted Muslim who knows the ritual. A coffin is not used unless the deceased was rich; rather, the body is carried in a cardboard box. Embalming and autopsies (unless court ordered) are prohibited. Muslims also reject cremation.

The body will usually be taken to a mosque, and an imam will lead the prayer for those who are present. The funeral happens at the cemetery; men are present, whereas women are discouraged from attending. Dignified mourning (weeping, but not loud wailing) is acceptable. Although it is best to bury the deceased within a day of the death, it is possible to delay it until the close family members can be present. In some Islamic denominations, special days of mourning are planned (e.g., third or seventh day after death, anniversary). A widow is not to interact with marriageable men for 4 months and 10 days after losing her husband to allow time for clarity about whether the deceased man has fathered a child, as well as to provide time for private grieving.

Role of Religious Community (Persons or Organizations) During Health Challenges

Regular congregational religious gatherings are conducted on Fridays, noon time, in mosques. The purposes for meeting are many: worship, community, meal, exchange of information, business (e.g., selling books, food). The worship involves a sermon and prayers, and attendees learn about how to incorporate the instructions of the *Qur'an* and *hadith* in daily life. In areas where there are a number of Muslims, there will be a local community social services network, usually associated with the mosque. An Islamic Center/Society/Community Association typically offers Muslims services such as religious education for children, scriptural study sessions for women and men, education for converts, services and resources for the sick and elders in the congregation, and Eid festivities.

Role of Clergy During Health Challenges

In Islamic societies, the clergy may function as both religious scholars and jurists. The clergy most likely to minister to the sick is the local mosque leader, the imam, who in Western societies, functions similarly as a priest and educated religious scholar. These religious leaders pray for those who are ill, comforting the sick and the family. Imams are usually available for home and hospital visits by arrangement.

Unique Religious Aspects of Family Involvement

Immediate family members (i.e., parents, children) will be those most integrally involved in caring for the sick. For example, it is family who can best offer prayers for the sick, and they also help to ritually cleanse the body of the deceased.

Nursing Implications Unique to This Religious Tradition

- Respecting the modesty of Muslim women is paramount. Keep their bodies covered as much as possible during nursing and medical procedures. If possible, offer male nurses to care for male patients and female nurses to attend to female Muslim patients.

- Praying is the basic ritual that a patient might desire when sick. Support patients to observe their daily prayers as requested by the patient. A basin with clean water may be brought to the bedside to allow the patient to make ablutions. If this is not possible, offering a pan with sand can substitute. The patient may also need assistance in being positioned so that his chest faces Mecca. A copy of the *Qur'an* (in Arabic or the patient's preferred language) may also be needed for prayer. A sick person may pray while sitting or lying in bed. If lying in bed, then position the bed so that the feet point to Mecca. The seriously ill and elderly who cannot pray are exempt from doing so. Although there are not gender differences in expectations about praying, it is recognized that not praying while menstruating is a mercy given to women.

- There are mercies prescribed for groups who may not be able to complete the fasts. The seriously ill, elderly, pregnant, and lactating women—those for whom it could be harmful, are exempt from the fast of

Ramadan. If Muslim patients are on medications and their condition is not life threatening, consider changing the timings of all medications to coincide between the sunset and sunrise to allow participation in fasting. All oral medications and fluids, any hydration or nutrition (including intravenous) will negate the fast.

• Muslims abstain from meat that has not been slaughtered properly or that has significant traces of blood. They also refrain from alcohol and pork products.

• The local Islamic organization or mosque can be contacted for resources or information. For example, if the family has not been able to identify a Muslim to assist with the ritual cleansing of the body of a deceased loved one, the nurse or chaplain can facilitate this request.

• For those preparing to pilgrimage to Mecca (*Hajj*), nurses can provide information and resources to address the potential health problems that can arise from prolonged exposure to millions of people and the desert environment (e.g., dehydration, communicable disease, foot care).

• The sick Muslim has a variety of scripturally based prescriptions for wellness. These include recitation of specific chapters of the *Quran*, drinking of *zam zam* (holy water sourced from Mecca), prayer, herbs, honey, and certain foods.

• If there are any issues with patients or families in a clinical setting (e.g., issues with prayers, fasting, traveling for Hajj), discuss with the people involved if they require support from their imam or a designated experienced, older Muslim woman who can offer support.

FOR MORE INFORMATION

View DVDs: *Islam: Empire of faith* (PBS), *Inside Islam* (History Channel), and *Inside Mecca* (National Geographic).

Visit http://www.metanexus.net/conferences/pdf/conference2006/Imam.pdf (for information about Islamic healing).

Denny, F. M. (2010). *An introduction to Islam* (4th ed.). Upper Saddle River, NJ: Prentice Hall.

Esposito, J. L. (1998). *Islam: The straight path.* New York, NY: Oxford University Press.

Gharaibeh, M. K., & Al Maaitah, R. (2011). Islam and nursing. In M. D. Fowler, S. Reimer-Kirkham, R. Sawatzky, & E. J. Taylor (Eds.), *Religion, religious ethics, and nursing* (pp. 229–249). New York, NY: Springer Publishing Company.

23 Orthodox Christians

CONTRIBUTOR: *The Reverend John Matusiak, MDiv*
NURSE REVIEWER: *Michael Hensley, RN*

Theology and Social History

The Orthodox Christian Church—also known as the Eastern Orthodox Church, Greek Orthodox Church, Russian Orthodox Church, Ukrainian Orthodox Church, Serbian Orthodox Church, Romanian Orthodox Church, and so forth—is a single, worldwide Church united in faith, sacraments, and worship. While it has no single administrative center, the Patriarch of Constantinople is the "first among equals" of the world's Orthodox Christian hierarchs and enjoys a "primacy of honor." In North America, like other faith traditions, one finds parishes that have a definite ethnic heritage alongside parishes that have no particular ethnic background. In fact, in North America, it is not uncommon to find converts to the faith that have no particular ethnic or national tradition. There are an estimated two million faithful in North America who worship in approximately 2,800 churches and mission communities, whereas worldwide, there are an estimated 200–300 million Orthodox Christians.

The Orthodox Christian Church traces its origin to the day of Pentecost, 50 days after Christ's Resurrection, when the Holy Spirit descended upon the apostles. Subsequently, five "patriarchates," or primary centers of Church life, were recognized: Rome, Constantinople, Alexandria, Antioch, and Jerusalem. In the mid-11th century, Rome formally broke communion with the other patriarchates, which remain in communion with one another to this day. Throughout its history, Orthodox Christianity has been missionary in nature, and today, it is found in virtually every corner of the world. Orthodox Christianity was planted in North America in 1794 with the arrival of missionaries from Russia in Kodiak, Alaska.

Ultimately, humans are created for communion with God in His everlasting Kingdom. Thus, central to Orthodox is the value placed on the Christian community. Although a personal relationship with Christ or the Holy Spirit is vital, this is not possible apart from the Christian community. The fundamental action of the People of God is to worship Father, Son, and Holy Spirit.

Deity/God or Ultimate Other

Orthodox Christianity is Trinitarian; that is, believers worship God the Father, God the Son (Jesus Christ, Who took on the human nature while retaining His divine nature as the Messiah and Savior), and God the Holy Spirit. Persons communicate with God primarily through formal public worship and private prayer, meditation and reflection, fasting, almsgiving, and acts of mercy and compassion (e.g., feeding the hungry, clothing the naked, ministering to the sick and imprisoned).

Views on Health and Well-Being

Being well is the default for the human nature; however, as a consequence of the sin of Adam and Eve, sickness and death became part of humankind's experience in this "fallen world."

Explanations for Disease and Illness

Modern scientific explanations for disease are accepted. Viewing disease or illness as punishment or the will of God are not congruent with Orthodox belief.

The Nature of Suffering and How to Address It

Suffering occurs when one's life is out of balance spiritually, physically, and emotionally, especially when one sees nothing greater than himself or herself. Though suffering is never something anyone wants in life, it is always assumed that good will come of it, thereby bringing comfort. "And we know that all things work together for good to them that love God . . ." (Romans 8:28). Maintaining spiritual health allows one to find such comfort.

Death, Dying, and Afterlife

Death is the parting of the soul from the body. Although Jesus Christ revealed that there is an afterlife, He revealed little detail. Having parted from the body, the soul remains conscious and alive so that at the end of time it will be reunited with the body in the "general resurrection" of the dead.

While planning how to comfort an Orthodox patient, one must consider his or her level of faith and relationship with God, family, and the faith community—or lack thereof.

Quick and Condensed Definitions of Terms

Orthodox—Commonly interpreted as correct believing.

Liturgy or Divine Liturgy—The primary public worship service celebrated every Sunday and on feast days and special occasions; involves prayers, reading of Scripture, Holy Communion.

Prayer

Simply stated, prayer is the conscious recollection that God is present with us at all times and in all places: He hears and assists us in our time of need and suffering; He is the Source of Life and Benefactor and Physician of our souls and bodies; He is to be praised and thanked in all things for His blessings; and His will must be discerned and accepted. Prayer involves far more than merely talking to God or asking God to fulfill our requests and wants.

Orthodox Christians are all called to pray for the sick and suffering, privately and in public worship. Likewise, prayers for the departed are offered at specific times, especially during the 40-day mourning period that follows death, in faithfulness to 1 Maccabees 19:39, "It is good to pray for the dead." How, precisely, our prayers affect the departed has not been revealed, however.

Religious Calendar

Sunday is the weekly holy day allowing believers to celebrate the resurrection of Jesus. Twelve feast days, in addition to Pascha (Easter), the Feast of Feasts, are on the Orthodox liturgical calendar. Special rituals, prayers, meals, and so forth are associated with many of these celebrations, the nature of which can vary from family to family, based on their background and heritage.

Health-Promoting Practices

The body is the "Tabernacle of the Holy Spirit." As such, it should not be put in a position that might cause it physical harm (e.g., smoking, excessive drinking, addictive drugs). Fasting, the refraining from eating meat, dairy products, and certain other foods on most Wednesdays and Fridays and the Church's Lenten season, is also observed with the conscious understanding that moderation in all things is healthful. Typically, fasts allow the eating of fruits, juices, steamed vegetables, nuts, bread, honey, and margarine. Christ Himself fasted, as revealed in Scripture. However, fasting is not practiced for health promotion; rather, it is an ascetic practice that allows for the development of self-discipline in all things. Those who are hospitalized or facing serious illness are exempt from the regular fasting regime. Indeed, depending on the health circumstances, fasting may not in itself be healthy.

Healing Rituals

The Sacrament of Holy Unction—during which anointing takes place—may be celebrated at any time, not just when death is imminent. Should death be imminent, the "Service for the Parting of the Soul from the Body" is celebrated. Some of the faithful may not be aware of these services, so it is critical that the patient's parish priest or others be contacted immediately upon learning of an illness.

Other Unique Religious Beliefs, Rites, and Practices Related to Health or Illness

In addition to that noted immediately above, the faithful generally requests vs request the sacraments of Confession and, especially, Holy Communion, "for the healing of soul and body and the remission of sins."

Unique Religious Beliefs, Rites, and Practices Related to Birthing

There are a variety of rites and practices surrounding birth: the Rite of the Naming of the Child on the Eighth Day after Birth, the Rite of Churching of the Mother and the Child, the Rite of Baptism, etc. These are, naturally, handled by the parish priest or other parish clergy and arranged between the family and the clergy.

Unique Religious Beliefs, Rites, or Practices Related to Childrearing

Baptism occurs when an infant is about 40 days old. The baptism, performed by a bishop or priest, involves full immersion three times in the name of the Father, Son, and Holy Spirit. In conjunction with baptism, a child (or adult, as the case may be) also receives the sacraments of Chrismation (the anointing/sealing with Holy Chrism that imparts the Gift of the Holy Spirit) and Holy Communion. Collectively, these are known as the "Rites of Initiation" and signify a new, spiritual birth into the life of Christ and His Body, the Church. In cases of emergency (e.g., imminent death of a newborn child), a family's parish priest should be contacted immediately. If clergy cannot be present, a layperson may baptize with water, "in the name of the Father, Son and Holy Spirit." Should the child survive, the remainder of the Rite, which includes Chrismation and Holy Communion, would be celebrated. Stillborn babies are not baptized. An Orthodox child will have godparents who agree to support the parents in spiritual instruction of the new Christian. In addition to the training from the parents and godparents, children and teens can receive Christian training at church and in Orthodox colleges and seminaries.

Unique Beliefs, Practices, and Rituals Surrounding Dying, Death, and Bereavement

The practices surrounding death can be quite complicated, depending on the patient, family traditions, and customs. Hence, it is essential that an Orthodox priest be contacted. Should death be imminent, the "Service for the Parting of the Soul from the Body" is celebrated by the priest. Various prayers and liturgies occur between death and burial. Special prayer services are celebrated on the 3rd, 9th, and 40th day after death occurs, as well as on the 6 month and annual anniversaries of death.

The body of the deceased is treated with the utmost respect as "the tabernacle of the Holy Spirit." No extraordinary means to prolong life should be undertaken; similarly, no extraordinary means to hasten death should be taken. Cremation is not sanctioned; burial is the norm.

Role of Religious Community (Persons or Organizations) During Health Challenges

A patient may participate in his or her parish worship and ministries to the extent he or she is able. Homebound individuals receive regular visits from his or her parish clergy and other parishioners. Many parishes have individuals who have been trained in visiting the sick. When a patient becomes ill or a family requires support, this is handled almost exclusively by the local priest and parish, which usually has a network in this regard. In places where there is a large Orthodox Christian population and multiple congregations, one often finds networks beyond the parish; in other places where this is not the case, the parish provides necessary networking and ministry.

Role of Clergy During Health Challenges

Orthodox Christians, at least those engaged in their faith, immediately contact their parish clergy when illness occurs and in the event of a serious change in health circumstances. The parish priest will be actively involved in pastoral ministry to the patient. In no instance should a hospital staff member, chaplain, or otherwise attempt to replace the ministry of the patient's parish priest. For example, non-Orthodox Christian clergy or chaplains should not insist that Orthodox Christian patients receive Communion or other ministrations from them, as is sometimes the case. Orthodox Christian clergy are always available and "on call."

Unique Religious Aspects of Family Involvement

An Orthodox Christian family that recently immigrated to the United States from another country may have different expectations and customs, often based on societal and cultural experience, than a seventh-generation American-born Orthodox Christian. The "rule of thumb" is to be respectful of a family's unique dynamics, to let them happen, and to work in harmony with a patient's parish priest and the network provided by his or her parish community, which is well equipped to handle sensitive matters within the appropriate cultural context.

Nursing Implications Unique to This Tradition

- Encourage the patient and his or her family to make and maintain contact with the patient's parish priest, other clergy, parish nurse, or other lay minister trained in this area. Non-Orthodox hospital chaplains should not impose themselves on an Orthodox Christian family or discourage them from contacting their clergy, but should interface with the Orthodox clergy.

- Avoid thinking in stereotypes. Not all Orthodox Christians are Greek or Russian. The vast majority of Orthodox Christians in the United States are American-born, having little or no connection to an "old country."

- Fasting practices (on most Wednesdays, Fridays, and the Church's Lenten seasons) are relaxed or eliminated entirely for those in poor health, depending on their circumstances. Parish clergy generally explain this to the family.

- When a patient requests it, or when death is imminent, space and time should be respected for Orthodox clergy to perform Holy Unction or other appropriate rites.

- The bodies of the deceased must be treated with utmost respect as "the tabernacle of the Holy Spirit." Should a priest not be present at the time of death, he should be informed immediately thereafter, according to the family's wishes.

- Orthodox patients who want to read the Scripture may prefer reading from the Epistles, Gospels, and Psalms. Study guides and Bible commentaries from the Orthodox church are available.

FOR MORE INFORMATION

Visit http://oca.org, particularly the pages titled "About Orthodox Christianity" and "The Orthodox Faith." Detailed information on Orthodox Christian doctrine, worship, Bible and Church history, and spirituality is presented.

24 Pentecostals

CONTRIBUTOR: *Thomson K. Mathew, DMin, EdD*

NURSE REVIEWER: *Carl Christensen, PhD, RN*

Theology and Social History

The modern Pentecostal movement, which is over a hundred years old, traces its roots to a Bible College in Topeka, Kansas, and a Mission House on Azusa Street in Los Angeles, California, where an unusual revival took place from 1906 to 1909. Pentecostalism is the fastest growing segment of Christianity globally, most of the growth taking place outside the United States. This movement consists of three major wings: (1) classical Pentecostal churches such as the Assemblies of God, Church of God (Cleveland), and the predominantly African American Church of God in Christ, (2) independent charismatic churches represented by many mega churches and TV preachers, and (3) mainline denominational church members who consider themselves charismatic because of an experience referred to as being "baptized in the Holy Spirit."

Their understanding of being filled with the Holy Spirit distinguishes Pentecostals from other Christians. Pentecostal Christians believe in an experience called the baptism in the Holy Spirit, which enables them to receive gifts of the Holy Spirit such as speaking in tongues, healing, miracles, and prophecy. Pentecostals' faith strongly contributes to their personal and social identity. For instance, some classical Pentecostals teach against wearing makeup, ornaments, and so forth, as part of their understanding of "holiness and separation from the world." Likewise, this personal encounter with the Holy Spirit prompts others to evangelize using the latest technologies and innovations. Pentecostals freely use religious vocabulary in their conversations as they are eager to share their faith with others. Pentecostals in significant numbers have migrated to America from India, and several countries of Africa and South/Central America. A noticeable number of Indian Pentecostal immigrants are nurses in American and Canadian hospitals.

Deity/God or Ultimate Other

As Christians, most Pentecostals are Trinitarians (believing that God revealed Himself as Father, Son, and the Holy Spirit). United Pentecostals, a classical Pentecostal denomination, is not Trinitarian. All Pentecostals believe in a God who is personally concerned about them and the world He created. He revealed Himself through Jesus Christ. Believers can communicate with God through prayer in Jesus' name. God answers the prayers and supplications of his children.

Views on Health and Well-Being

Based on a word used by Jesus when he healed the sick, the Pentecostals define health as "wholeness," which is interpreted as being well in body, mind, and spirit. Some would extend this definition to include wellness of finances, relationships, and so forth. One of the benefits of the death of Jesus on the cross is physical healing. Pentecostals often quote Isaiah 53:5: "By His stripes we are healed."Additionally, the gifts of the Holy Spirit include healing, and as Spirit-filled people, they expect this gift to "manifest" in their lives. Healing is also expected as "signs and wonders" that follow the preaching of the word of God to confirm the word preached.

The major characteristic of all Pentecostals is their belief in speaking in tongues and some form of divine healing. Most Pentecostals are open to medical care, although some may feel that accepting medical care is an expression of lack of faith. A few in the very fringe of the movement may decline medical care due to this reason.

Explanations for Disease and Illness

Although some members of the community may consider illness as punishment for particular sins and use examples such as the connection between smoking and cancer, drinking and liver cirrhosis, most Pentecostals are comfortable believing that sickness is the result of human sinfulness in a fallen world. Adam's sin brought sickness and death into the world.

The Nature of Suffering and How to Address It

Pentecostals do not have a unified theology of suffering. While some in the charismatic wing believe that suffering has no place in a believer's life because Jesus once and for all took our suffering upon himself, others may believe that God is punishing people or chastening his children through suffering. Most will accept the mystery of suffering.

Death, Dying, and Afterlife

Pentecostals believe in life after death. They believe that only born again persons will go to heaven. They also believe in a literal hell. For a believer, to be absent from the body is to be present with Christ. They hope to be reunited with their loved ones in heaven. They expect the bodily resurrection of all believers at the second coming of Christ. Many believe that they will rule the earth for 1000 years on earth with Christ. There are strong disagreements within the community about the timing and sequence of these events. Seeing Jesus face to face is a comforting thought to the Pentecostals. They expect to receive certain rewards from Him. The concern of some patients would be the fate of loved ones who died without faith in Christ.

Quick and Condensed Definitions of Terms

Speaking in tongues—The phenomenon of speaking in an unlearned and unknown language believed to be empowered by the Holy Spirit; the Charismatic wing of the Pentecostal movement also calls this "prayer language" or "praying in the Spirit" (Acts 2:4).

Anointing oil—Oil (usually olive oil) used to anoint (touch with a drop) the sick as part of the prayer for healing (James 5:14).

Signs and Wonders—Miraculous occurrences, especially supernatural healing (Acts 5:12).

Born again—Inviting Jesus (his spirit, words, salvation, lordship, and eternal nature) into one's being (1 Peter 1:23).

Prayer

Prayer is vital to the Pentecostals. Prayer can be individual and/or corporate. It is not uncommon to see a group gathered around the patient's bed and praying in a rather loud voice or with hands raised. Clergy and laity will pray for the sick in their presence. People will often join hands as they pray. An elder may anoint the patient with oil at this time. (Typically, a minister will draw a cross on the patient's forehead with oil. Patients may also place on their person a handkerchief or another object anointed or prayed over by a minister.)

Religious Calendar

Pentecostals are not very sacramental in their religious practice. Although Easter and Christmas are important days, they do not have any special required observances attached to them.

Health-Promoting Practices

There are no required dietary practices. Members may fast and pray from time to time at their own discretion.

Healing Rituals

Patients may expect or request a visit from their clergy. Patients may ask visitors or even staff to pray for them. They may also call prayer groups in their churches. Daily reading of the Bible is normal for many. Some may listen to the Bible from recordings or find inspiration in listening to Christian music. They may watch religious programs on television.

Other Unique Religious Beliefs, Rites, and Practices Related to Health or Illness

Patients may report seeing visions or dreams. Some may report seeing Jesus or an angel in the room. They may say God spoke to them.

Unique Religious Beliefs, Rites, and Practices Related to Birthing

There are no specific observations. They do not baptize infants.

Unique Religious Beliefs, Rites, or Practices Related to Childrearing

There are no unique beliefs, rites, or practices.

Unique Beliefs, Practices, and Rituals Surrounding Dying, Death, and Bereavement

There are no specific religious practices. There may be ethnic and cultural variations with religious implications.

Role of Religious Community (Persons or Organizations) During Health Challenges

Pentecostals worship regularly on Sundays. They may attend worship or church-related activities during the week. They normally gather for worship in denominationally affiliated or independent churches. Individuals must confess their personal faith before baptism. Communion is observed on a regular basis, normally once a month in the United States.

There are no specific programs, but local churches and television ministries may reach out to patients based on their prior relationship with them. Many churches have trained volunteers who visit the sick. Local churches have varying levels of benevolence ministries.

Role of Clergy During Health Challenges

Pastors are licensed or ordained persons. They are expected to visit the sick. Clergy may bring communion to the patient upon request.

Unique Religious Aspects of Family Involvement

There are no unique aspects. Loved ones may fast and pray for a patient.

Nursing Implications Unique to this Religious Tradition

- Pentecostal patients and families may ask a nurse they trust to pray with them; an offer of prayer from a nurse is likely to be warmly received (e.g., "Would a prayer be helpful now?").

- A patient speaking in tongues is not necessarily a patient with a mental or language difficulty. Respect this prayer language as communion with God.

- Patients with distress-causing illness models (e.g., my illness is a punishment) may benefit from expert spiritual counseling that helps them to view illness/tragedy more positively (e.g., as mystery or opportunity to go deeper in their relationship with God). Make a referral to a certified chaplain or pastoral counselor if the patient consents.

- Pentecostals may want to express joy and celebrate something good that happens (e.g., birth, healing). The theistic nurse can offer an affirming comment like, "Yes, I praise God with you for this blessing."

FOR MORE INFORMATION

Visit the Assemblies of God website at www.ag.org.

Mathew, T. K. (2002). *Ministry between miracles: Caring for hurting people in the power of the Holy Spirit.* Fairfax, VA: Xulon Press.

Roberts, O. (1957). *If you need healing do these things.* Tulsa, Oklahoma: Oral Roberts Evangelistic Association.

Synan, V. (2001). *The century of the Holy Spirit.* Nashville, TN: Thomas Nelson Publishers.

25 Presbyterians and Others in the Reformed Tradition

CONTRIBUTOR: *The Reverend Marsha D. M. Fowler, PhD, MDiv, MS, FAAN*

NURSE REVIEWER: *Marilyn Halstead, PhD, RN*

Theology and Social History

The Reformed family of churches descends from the Swiss segment of the Protestant Reformation of the 1500 and 1600s. The Reformed churches spread throughout Europe, then to the United States through both Dutch Reformed and Scots Presbyterian immigrants and to other countries. Three sources of authority for the church include the Bible, the historic Creeds and Confessions, and the Constitution of the church (variously called the Book of Order, the Book of Church Order, Book of Common Order). There is agreement across Reformed churches internationally as to the theological distinctives of the Reformed Tradition. They are:

> Central to this tradition is the affirmation of the majesty, holiness, and providence of God, who creates, sustains, rules, and redeems the world in the freedom of sovereign righteousness and love. Related to this central affirmation of God's sovereignty are other great themes of the Reformed Tradition: (1) The election of the people of God for service as well as for salvation; (2) Covenant life marked by a disciplined concern for order in the church according to the Word of God; (3) A faithful stewardship that shuns ostentation and seeks proper use of the gifts of God's creation; (4) The recognition of the human tendency to idolatry and tyranny, which calls the people of God to work for the transformation of society by seeking justice and living in obedience to the Word of God. (Presbyterian Church [USA] Book of Order §G-2.0500)

Reformed Christians believe that, as followers of Jesus Christ, they are responsible for "speaking truth to power" and for uncovering "tyrannies and idolatries," whether in culture or the church itself. Those in the Reformed tradition join the struggle for justice for all, especially for poor and vulnerable persons or groups, and work to create ministries of compassion for the poor, the sick, the refugee, the dispossessed, and disenfranchised. Reformed Christians have propounded a strong doctrine of "vocation," affirming that whatever the work (e.g., nursing) in which one is engaged, if one obeys one's calling in it, it should be understood as a calling from God to serve God's glory, our joy, and neighbor's good.

Reformed churches are predominantly Presbyterian in polity, where the congregation is governed by a group of elected elders who are lay persons and a minister. Regional groups of churches form a *Presbytery*, and groups of *Presbyteries* form *Synods* that together form the national General Assembly. Great emphasis is placed upon having an educated clergy as well as an educated laity. In the United States (and also elsewhere in the world), Presbyterians differ somewhat from the general population in that over 60% have a college degree, compared with less than 25% of the general population.

Deity/God or Ultimate Other

The Reformed Tradition is monotheistic, affirming one God, in three persons (i.e., Holy Trinity). The persons of the Trinity are God the Father, God the Son (made incarnate, that is becoming human, in Jesus the Christ), and God the Holy Spirit (or, in older terminology, the Holy Ghost). God is one in substance. God is holy, omniscient, omnipotent, omnipresent, uncreated, infinite, spirit, loving, just, merciful, and seeks communion with humankind and growth in righteousness of followers.

God is concerned for the personal lives of all and intervenes on behalf of humankind. God is God-for-us. Individuals and groups communicate with God through prayer, contemplation, and meditation. God responds to humankind in many ways and is self-revealing through the Bible, the holy scriptures of the Christian Church. Those scriptures include the Jewish Scriptures (*Tanach*) and the New Testament. God's Holy Spirit leads and guides believers through a variety of means (e.g., Scripture, wise counsel, pastoral care). When the individual claims to be led by God, the "test" for God's guidance is its conformity to scripture and its validation by the community of faith.

Views on Health and Well-Being

Health and well-being are defined in both individual and social terms. Human life is lived within a world that has suffered from human willfulness (disobedience to God); the consequence of this has been misery and injustice throughout human history. Believers recognize their finitude and imperfection and the unreachability of wholeness apart from God. Healing and health, then, reside within human efforts toward wholeness for one and all; that is, in obedience to God, people ameliorate and eradicate the causes of misery, injustice, and all that which damages human flourishing. Reformed Christians are called, always and everywhere, to a committed pursuit of social justice and human wholeness.

Explanations for Disease and Illness

Disease, illness, suffering, and death, and indeed natural disaster as well, are a consequence of humankind's choosing to go its own way and to live independent of God (called "sin"). Human sin brings about "The Fall" wherein humankind falls away from God and from God's unmerited favor (grace). Although humanity remains prone to tyranny and idolatry (sin)—that is, to choosing wrongly, God loves humankind even so. The consequence of human sinfulness in the Fall is that the created world is, itself, broken and fallen and in need of redemption and healing. Disease, illness, suffering, and death are ultimately a consequence of the Fall and afflicts both "the just, and the unjust."

The Nature of Suffering and How to Address It

Suffering is an inevitable part of the human condition and the lot of all humans: all will suffer in this life. However, we are not alone in our suffering, for our loving God walks with us in our suffering and comforts and cares for us ("Yea, though I walk through the valley of the shadow of death, I will fear no evil for Thou art with me . . ." Bible, Psalm 23).

Death, Dying, and Afterlife

Theologically, death is a consequence of human willfulness or going our own way in disobedience to God. Reformed Christians do believe in an afterlife in the presence of God in which there will be neither sickness nor sorrow. Life itself is a gift and a loan from God, and we are to steward it and preserve it as we are able. Yet life is not to be preserved at any or all costs; life is not a second God.

Quick and Condensed Definitions of Terms

Reformed Christian religious terminology reflects, in large part, that found in mainstream Protestant Christian traditions.

Prayer

Prayer is a means of communication with God and may be individual, group, or corporate. It may be: free prayer (without form or specific words, praying as one is led to pray); form prayer (where the structure or format of the prayer is set but the content is not); or set prayer (where the words of the prayer are "set," for example, the Lord's Prayer). Members of the Reformed Tradition are expected to pray for one another both individually and as a part of the worship service. Religious leaders do pray for "ordinary" members in their own private prayers, in prayer with the individual, in prayer groups, and in the worship service. Churches often have a "prayer chain" that is a group of individuals who are notified of a need for prayer and who are contacted for immediate prayer. Prayer may be for individuals who participate in the life of the congregation, for those known to the congregation or its members (but not members), for those who suffer (e.g., local, national, or international disaster), for enduring world problems (e.g., peace in the Middle East), or for groups of individuals who are in need (e.g., unemployed persons, homeless persons). While the faithful may pray for miracles of healing, they understand that such unusual intervention is God's choice and that God's loving presence with and among us is in itself a miracle.

Religious Calendar

With all Christian liturgical churches, the Reformed Tradition observes the liturgical cycle of the Christian year. The most important days of the year include Easter, Christmas, Pentecost, Ash Wednesday, Maundy Thursday, Good Friday, Epiphany, Reformation Sunday, and more. These holy days will be marked by worship services. On holy days that are festivals (e.g., Pentecost), there may be a celebration after worship that includes a lunch, cake, and so forth. In the Reformed and other Christian traditions, there is customarily a family gathering and meal on Christmas and Easter.

Health-Promoting Practices

The Reformed Tradition does not specify specific practices that are either prescribed or proscribed. Rather, we are to remember that our lives are not our own, and we are to be good stewards of life. That means that we are to use the means of God's good creation (i.e., human intelligence, knowledge, skill, wisdom—research, science) in our pursuit of health for ourselves and for our society.

Healing Rituals

We offer "anointing with oil" for any and all those who are ill or in need of healing. This may be done for individuals, groups, or congregations. There are liturgies for a worship and prayer service of healing and wholeness that can be offered for congregations. We also use "laying on of hands" (a hand of blessing upon the head or shoulder) by religious leaders, which is always accompanied by prayer.

Other Unique Religious Beliefs, Rites, and Practices Related to Health or Illness

The rites, rituals, and practices of the Reformed Tradition are shared among almost all Christian traditions.

Unique Religious Beliefs, Rites, and Practices Related to Birthing

There are no unique religious beliefs, rites, or practices surrounding childbirth. Infants in danger of death are not customarily baptized unless it pastorally serves to comfort the parents. Baptism is not theologically required or essential for a dying infant. Circumcision of male infants is a parental choice that has no religious implications.

Unique Religious Beliefs, Rites, or Practices Related to Childrearing

Children, as in all Christian traditions, are to be reared "in the nurture and admonition of the Lord," to be educated in the faith (usually through Sunday School and Vacation Bible School), to be taught to read the Bible, and to learn the polity and beliefs distinctive of the Reformed Tradition. Children are baptized as infants and customarily take their first communion when they can understand its meaning. In the United States, they are "confirmed" in the faith and enter into church membership (formally, on their own) and receive a copy of the Bible from the elders of the congregation customarily sometime between age 8 and high school.

Unique Beliefs, Practices, and Rituals Surrounding Dying, Death, and Bereavement

As in all Christian traditions, members are cared for spiritually by the pastor and deacons and other members of the congregation in their dying days and surrounding death. Bereavement care is customarily the responsibility of the pastor of the congregation. A funeral or memorial service (that is a worship service that takes account of and celebrates the life of the person who has died) is conducted. A funeral in which the body of the deceased person is present takes place usually within 3 days of the death. A memorial service (when the body is not present) takes place anytime after the death, but usually within 1 to 2 weeks. The funeral or memorial service is most frequently held in the church itself, though this is not a requirement. There is, additionally, a brief graveside service when the body or ashes are interred. A memorial or funeral service will include prayer, hymns, eulogies, scripture reading, and a brief sermon. A graveside service will include prayers, perhaps singing, recitation of scripture, and committal of the person to God. The Reformed Tradition has no religious specifications regarding the preparation of the body, burial over cremation, or the time at which the body must be interred. Bereavement care is given to the family but may also be given to the congregation that is grieving the loss of a beloved member.

Role of Religious Community (Persons or Organizations) During Health Challenges

In the Reformed Tradition, congregations hold worship services every Sunday and on holy days that do not fall on Sundays. The main practices and rituals in these gatherings for corporate worship include prayer (pastoral prayer, liturgical prayer, and prayers of the people), corporate

confession of sin, hymn singing, reading of the scriptures, and the proc-
lamation of the scriptures (preaching a "sermon"). These worship services may at times include a baptism or the Lord's Supper, also known
as Communion or the Eucharist. Additional worship services are held
for special occasions or needs such as services of healing and wholeness,
dedication of a church building, weddings, and funerals (which are to
be services of worship). Reformed congregations also gather for meals,
celebrations of many types (e.g., a member's 50th wedding anniversary),
for Sunday School (adult and child Christian education), and for "officer
training" (elder and deacon training).

Some congregations have a parish nurse or Stephen's ministry, though
these are not unique to the Reformed or Protestant tradition. Although
there are no organizations, as such, that care for the sick, Deacons assume
this role. Every congregation has a group of persons, called "deacons,"
who are elected and ordained to a ministry of comfort, compassion, and
witness. "The office of deacon as set forth in Scripture is one of compassion, witness, and service after the example of Jesus Christ. Persons of
spiritual character, honest repute, of exemplary lives, brotherly and sis-
terly love, sincere compassion, and sound judgment should be chosen for
this office . . . . It is the duty of deacons, first of all, to minister to those who
are in need, to the sick, to the friendless, and to any who may be in distress
both within and beyond the community of faith" (§G-6.0402).

Reformed congregations draw upon social services offered in local
communities to meet needs not addressed by individual congregations.
That is to say, local congregations do not duplicate services being offered
in the community. However, Presbyterian denominations have a variety of
social service agencies, active in cooperation with other religious and civil
agencies, that respond to any major emergency or disaster worldwide (e.g.,
earthquake, wildfire, hurricane, nuclear disaster, epidemic) with immediate financial and material resource assistance. This assistance is provided
without regard for religious preference or affiliation of the recipients.

Role of Clergy During Health Challenges

Members of the congregation (whether an official member or not) should
expect hospital visits by the pastor (and possibly a deacon, or an elder as
well). The pastor (also called a "minister" or "teaching elder") is responsible for visiting the ill, for attending the dying, for conducting funeral and
memorial services, and for comforting the bereaved. The pastor also leads
the community in prayer for those who are ill, dying, suffering, grieving,
or in need. In many instances, the pastor will anoint with oil those who
are ill and pray with them. Pastors may also conduct worship services of
"healing and wholeness" for a whole congregation where those who are
suffering, ill, in crisis, or in need may receive special prayer, anointing,
and "laying on of hands."

Unique Religious Aspects of Family Involvement

There are no unique aspects of family involvement in the Reformed tradition. As with other religious persons, family members may pray with and for the person who is ill.

Nursing Implications Unique to This Religious Tradition

- There are no specific or direct implications for nursing practice that are unique to the Reformed tradition that are not common to other Christian tradition (e.g., sense of guilt or remorse requiring referral to clergy or desire for prayer with others).

- Those patients who are accustomed to regular church attendance may wish to have copies of the sermon or to receive communion or anointing in the hospital. If they are aware of the hospitalization, however, the pastor and deacon or elder will have visited the patient and have ascertained their religious needs.

FOR MORE INFORMATION

Visit the Christian Reformed Church of North America's website (especially Beliefs section) www.crcna.org, Reformed Church of America (www.rca.org), Presbyterian Church in America (www.pcaac.org), and General Assembly Mission Council of the Presbyterian Church (USA) at http://gamc.pcusa.org/ministries/phewa/who-we-are. These websites offer information about doctrines, church history, and position papers of relevance to nurses.

Vaux, K. (1984). *Health and medicine in the reformed tradition*. New York, NY: Crossroad.

26 Roman Catholics

CONTRIBUTOR: *Father Luke Dysinger, OSB, MD, DPhil*

NURSE REVIEWER: *Denise Miner-Williams, PhD, RN, CHPN*

Theology and Social History

Roman Catholicism is the continuation of Christianity practiced in Western Europe from the first through the sixteenth centuries. Catholics acknowledge the Pope (the Bishop of Rome) as leader of the Church with authority to define Catholic doctrine and appoint bishops who oversee dioceses (large geographic regions that sometimes correspond to county or state boundaries). The religious turmoil of the 16th century created numerous independent "protestant" Christian denominations that do not acknowledge the authority of the Pope. However, the Catholic Church remains the largest branch of Christianity, with over 1.1 billion members worldwide. The Catholic Church in North America is extremely diverse, culturally, socially, and politically. The majority of Catholics are of Western European, Hispanic, or Asian descent and worship according to the Latin or "Western" rite, using modern translations of ancient Latin prayers and ceremonies. However, there also exist smaller communities of "Eastern Rite Catholics" whose worship and practices reflect Greek, Russian, and Near-Eastern traditions.

Immigration, with its attendant opportunities and disadvantages, continues to play an important role in the growth and social makeup of all U.S. Catholic parishes (local congregations). Parishes vary a great deal in size. In large urban centers, parishes may be very large. For example, an average-sized parish in the Archdiocese of Los Angeles may comprise more than 3,000 families. Within each parish, there are frequently cultural subgroups, often with designated "Masses" (worship services, see "Role of Religious Community" on page 247) in their own language. In most dioceses in North America, ordinations to the priesthood are insufficient to provide for the pastoral needs of Catholic communities, especially in regions such as the American Southwest where the Catholic Church is steadily growing in numbers. Catholic parishes are thus frequently understaffed, with only a few priests (usually one to three, often only one) and a variable number of lay ministers serving their sometimes very large and diverse communities.

Deity/God or Ultimate Other

Roman Catholicism is theistic. God is described as the Blessed Trinity, "One God in Three Persons, Father, Son, and Holy Spirit" (The Catechism of the Catholic Church [CCC], 249–256). This means that God is regarded as the creator and sustainer of the universe, active in all natural and human affairs, capable of intervening both through miracles (events that seem to be or actually are independent of natural laws) and in ordinary events. God became a human being in the historical person of Jesus Christ whose example, teachings, and redeeming death, make it possible for all humans to be saved from selfishness, sin, and death and to live forever with God in heaven. The Holy Spirit is the Person of the Trinity who comes to people as a teacher of the meaning of God, who fills them with the power and grace to understand, and who puts courage in their hearts to witness and live what is believed.

Catholics experience God chiefly through prayer, sacramental worship, reading of the Bible or other spiritual texts, meditation, and charitable deeds. Community worship is an important aspect of living the Catholic faith. Charitable deeds, or compassionate actions toward one's neighbor, afford an opportunity to both cooperate with God's will and to contemplate the presence of God in others.

Views on Health and Well-Being

Roman Catholics believe that mind, body, and spirit comprise a unity. Thus, "health" exists when the different facets of the self are in balance and harmony. Physical and psychological health, as they are understood by modern medicine, are important elements in this harmony. But equally important are the dimensions of conscience, will, and spirit: that is, the ability to appreciate the significance of moral choices, the freedom to act in accordance with God's will, and the decision to commune with God through prayer and worship. Thus, when physical and psychological health decline—as natural life draws to its end, the human person can maintain spiritual health by remaining oriented toward God.

Explanations for Disease and Illness

The Catholic Church relies on science to describe the biological causes of disease and illness. When patients ask for a spiritual or metaphysical explanation of the cause of their disease, any attempt at an answer will be at best partial and should always be offered in a spirit of profound humility and loving compassion. How the existence of disease can be reconciled with faith in a loving God is a mystery that has never been satisfactorily answered. Although illness and death are in some way associated with human sinfulness, patients should never regard their own illness as a specific punishment from God for their sins. Instead, they should be encouraged to seek consolation and meaning through prayer and meditation on the example of Christ who has a "preferential love" for the sick and who gives meaning to all suffering and illness.

The Nature of Suffering and How to Address It

God does not will that humans should suffer; rather, God is present in all pain and will help those who search for the meaning and purpose of their suffering. All suffering has been given value and meaning by Jesus' death on the cross, but such meaning can never be imposed from without by others who are not themselves in pain. Thus, unless they are specifically asked to do so, a priest, minister, or health care worker should not try to impose on the sick their own interpretation of the meaning of that patient's suffering. Instead, they should listen, support, and pray for the patient, encouraging the person to pray and seek answers from God. In time, the patient may be able to share with them a sense of what their suffering means.

Death, Dying, and Afterlife

Death is the gateway to eternal life. Christians will find that the love of Jesus Christ that they experience in prayer and the sacraments will deepen and become eternal in the joyful embrace of Heaven, where they will enjoy communion with God and all the saved. Catholics believe that salvation is possible for people who are ignorant of Christ and His Church: those who "seek the truth and do the will of God in accordance with their understanding of it, can be saved" (CCC, 1260). However, those who prefer isolation and reject communion with God will discover in death the power of freely choosing "definitive self-exclusion from God and the blest" (CCC, 1033). Heaven is sometimes described as the vision of God's face. The sick and dying may take comfort in the Catholic teaching that the purification that makes beatific vision possible need not be complete by the time of a person's death: it will continue and be brought to fruition in the "world to come" (CCC, 1030).

Quick and Condensed Definitions of Terms

Clergy—Ministers (only men) officially ordained by a Catholic bishop. Three orders of clergy include:

> *Bishop*—The leader and highest authority within a diocese (designated geographical region); can perform all rites and celebrate all sacraments.

> *Priest*—Ordained; able to celebrate all sacraments except ordination. Only priests and bishops may hear confessions, celebrate Mass, and anoint the sick. Deacons and lay chaplains may not perform these

rites. The priest in charge of a parish is known as "the Pastor" and may be assisted by one or more associate priests, sometimes called "parochial vicars."

Deacon—Ordained Catholic minister able to preach, preside at baptisms, and weddings. Deacons may be married when ordained, but may not marry after being ordained.

Sacraments—Religious ceremonies considered to confer special grace. The seven sacraments of the Catholic Church are Baptism, Confirmation, The Eucharist, Penance and Reconciliation, The Anointing of the Sick, Holy Orders (Ordination), and Matrimony.

Prayer

Prayer is "the raising of one's mind and heart to God or the requesting of good things from God" (CCC, 2259). Everyone is encouraged to pray frequently, honestly, and simply, according to the example of Jesus, who particularly recommended the "Our Father" as a formula for prayer. Prayer is frequently offered in community, but Catholics are also encouraged to set aside time for private prayer, particular on arising in the morning, before meals, and before going to sleep. Catholics are encouraged to pray for and to request the prayers of both the living and the deceased, especially "saints," whose lives are considered to have been particularly exemplary of Christian virtue.

All Catholics are expected to pray for the sick, both those whom they know personally and those unknown to them. The names of the sick are often recited during public worship and are sometimes published in Sunday parish bulletins and newsletters. Most parishes have a secretary who coordinates this information and who will be grateful to receive the name of hospitalized Catholics from that parish, so they may be remembered in the community's prayers. Prayer for the sick (like all prayer) may be offered in community or privately; it may be spontaneous or "liturgical" that is offered according to a set form, often a series of responses by individuals in a group. Prayers for the sick and the deceased sometimes take the form of Masses celebrated for that person's intention and remembrance.

Priests and lay Catholic chaplains in hospitals always prefer to pray in the presence of the sick, whether the individual is conscious or not. Such prayer is often liturgical, following the form prescribed in ritual texts. Catholics participate in such prayers by offering brief, formulaic responses, and many may be uncomfortable if they are expected to offer spontaneous prayers of their own.

Religious Calendar

Catholics who are able to attend Mass are expected to do so on Sundays and "days of obligation" including Christmas (December 25), All Saints

(November 1), the Feasts of the Assumption (August 15), and Immaculate Conception (December 7) of the Blessed Virgin Mary. The number of days of obligation varies in different countries and dioceses. The sick are exempt from this requirement, although if at all possible, they should be offered the opportunity to receive Holy Communion on Sundays and major feasts. Various Catholic subcultures attach additional importance to certain feasts and celebrations, such as the Feast of Our Lady of Guadalupe (December 12) for Hispanics. Ash Wednesday (the beginning of the penitential season of Lent, 46 days before Easter) is an important day when prayer, fasting, and almsgiving are particularly encouraged, and Catholics receive special ashes on their foreheads as a sign of repentance. Ashes may be distributed by authorized laypersons and should be offered to the sick.

Health-Promoting Practices

Fasting (limiting food to one full meal per day) and abstinence from meat is required of Catholics in good health between the ages of 14 and 60 on Ash Wednesday and Good Friday (the Friday before Easter) and abstinence from meat on the Fridays of Lent. In some countries and dioceses, abstinence from meat is required on all Fridays throughout the year.

Healing Rituals

The Catholic Church provides a rich variety of ceremonies, sacramental rituals, and prayers that should be made available to the sick. Of the following, the first two are sacraments that may only be celebrated by a Catholic priest or bishop: The Sacrament of Penance and Reconciliation ("Confession") allows one to confess to God in the hearing of the priest all serious sins committed since the last confession. Absolution (forgiveness) is pronounced, and the patient is encouraged to offer a prayer or perform some simple act of "penance" as a sign of sorrow for sin. Anything confessed to the priest is held in absolute confidence and may not be divulged to anyone for any reason.

The Anointing of the Sick (formerly called "Extreme Unction") is administered to anyone with a serious illness or who faces surgery. It should not be delayed until the patient is terminally ill or near death. It may be repeated if the patient's condition significantly worsens. The elderly may be anointed if they are in weak condition even though no dangerous illness is present. The patient is anointed on the forehead and hands with blessed olive oil while prayers are offered. This sacrament effects spiritual healing and forgiveness of sins. It may be administered to unconscious or incompetent patients who could reasonably be presumed to request it if they were able.

Although Mass may only be celebrated by a Catholic priest, the bread consecrated at Mass ("The Host" or "Holy Communion") may be brought to the sick by designated lay ministers. The Sacrament of Holy Baptism, which initiates an individual into membership in the Catholic Church, may occasionally be requested by a dying patient or the parents of a seriously ill infant. In an emergency when a Catholic priest is unavailable, baptism may be administered by anyone, regardless of their religious beliefs, whose intention is to baptize the patient according to the beliefs and practice of the Catholic Church. The sacrament consists of pouring water three times on the head of the patient while saying "I baptize you in the name of the Father, and of the Son, and of the Holy Spirit. Amen." The local Catholic parish should be notified of any emergency baptisms so they can be recorded in the parish register.

Other Unique Religious Beliefs, Rites, and Practices Related to Health or Illness

Many Catholics attach importance to religious pictures (e.g., holy cards) or images (e.g., crucifix or statues), or the rosary (a circle of beads used in a ritual of prayers) and may wish to keep these near their bedside or on their person. Where these wishes can reasonably be accommodated, it may provide great comfort and reassurance to the patient. During some Catholic rituals, it is customary to sprinkle blessed water in the room or on the sick person. If this is contraindicated, the patient and family should be informed of this.

Unique Religious Beliefs, Rites, and Practices Related to Birthing

Catholics believe that abortion (intentionally destroying the life an unborn child) is always wrong, even when it is medically recommended to safeguard the mother's health. An emergency baptism of a dying infant (or person of any age) may be administered by any person who is properly disposed (see "Healing Rituals").

Unique Religious Beliefs, Rites, or Practices Related to Childrearing

Parents are ultimately responsible for the formation of their children's faith, but they supplement their home teaching and practices with formal religious education classes, also called faith formation or CCD (Confraternity of Christian Doctrine, or Catechism). These organized classes are offered at pre-K through high school level and are often required for sacramental preparation (for first Holy Eucharist [Communion], Reconciliation, and Confirmation). Children attending Catholic schools have this learning incorporated within the curriculum and therefore do not attend CCD classes.

Unique Beliefs, Practices, and Rituals Surrounding Dying, Death, and Bereavement

Sacramental ministry to the dying should include, if possible, the Sacraments of Penance and Reconciliation, Anointing of the Sick, and Holy Communion (see "Healing Rituals"). When Holy Communion is offered to the dying, it is called "viaticum." These sacraments should be provided only if the patient is still living. If the patient has died (e.g., declared brain dead), sacraments should not be administered. Prayers for the deceased, however, should be said, and Masses may be offered for that person's intention and remembrance.

Euthanasia is considered morally unacceptable and a serious violation of God's law as it is considered not to eliminate suffering but rather the person who suffers (John Paul II, Egvangelium Vitae, 65). Catholics on the other hand, however, are not obliged to consent to treatment that will only serve to prolong the process of dying and cause undue suffering. Despite misunderstandings and frequent reluctance based on cultural traditions, for Catholics "organ donation after death is a noble and meritorious act and is to be encouraged as an expression of generous solidarity" (CCC, 2296).

Role of Religious Community (Persons or Organizations) During Health Challenges

Communal worship is an integral aspect of Catholicism. The central and most important Catholic religious ceremony is the celebration of Mass, also called "The Eucharist." This ceremony consists of a "penitential rite" including a corporate confession of sin and prayer for absolution; set readings from the Bible followed by a sermon-commentary on the readings; prayers of intercession for particular needs and persons; and a partial re-enactment of Jesus' final Passover celebration with His disciples, including the "Words of Consecration" that are believed by Catholics to transform bread and wine into the Body and Blood of Jesus, which is then consumed by worshippers as Holy Communion. Participating in Sunday Mass is a requirement, and in addition, daily Mass attendance is important to many devout Catholics.

Ideally, if the hospital has a chapel and a Catholic chaplain or visiting priest, patients may be transported to the chapel and participate fully in the liturgy of the Mass. Where this is not possible, Holy Communion (the consecrated host) may be brought to the sick by Catholic lay ministers, who will pray with the sick person some of the prayers of the Mass. Those who care for the sick can be of great help by arranging the schedule so as to allow the sick person time to both receive Holy Communion and to meditate in silence for a brief time afterward.

There are a large number of Catholic religious orders and societies dedicated to the care of the sick and the poor, such as the Missionaries of Charity, the Daughters of Charity, the Brothers of St. John of God, and the Society of St. Vincent de Paul. Contact information for these and other Catholic agencies can be obtained from the local Catholic diocesan office (sometimes called the "chancery"). Most parishes provide training programs for lay persons who are specially commissioned to visit and minister to the sick, especially by bringing them Holy Communion. They can be contacted through the local Catholic parish.

Role of Clergy During Health Challenges

Parish priests normally arrange for the spiritual care of sick members of their parish, either by visiting them personally or by arranging for them to be visited by chaplains or lay ministers.

Unique Religious Aspects of Family Involvement

This varies considerably, depending on cultural traditions. Most Catholic families "rally to the bedside" of seriously ill family members. Family members are generally encouraged to take part in prayers and sacramental ministry to the sick. Given how it is often difficult to obtain consensus from an emotionally distraught family, advance directives should be encouraged whenever possible.

Nursing Implications Unique to This Religious Tradition

- Catholics often participate in recited prayers or by offering brief, formulaic responses to a prayer and may be uncomfortable if they are expected to offer spontaneous prayers of their own.

- Fasting (limiting food to one full meal per day) and abstinence from meat is required of Catholics in good health between the ages of 14 and 60 on Ash Wednesday and Good Friday (the Friday before Easter) and abstinence from meat on the Fridays of Lent. In some countries and dioceses, abstinence from meat is required on all Fridays throughout the year. The sick are exempt if fasting is deleterious to their health.

- Catholics should be offered the opportunity to receive Holy Communion on Sundays and major feasts—at the bedside with the support of a lay minister or at a chapel Mass if available. Likewise, on Ash Wednesdays, the ashes can be received on the Catholic patient's forehead. Nurses can plan patients' schedules not only to allow time for Holy Communion but also time to meditate in silence for a brief time afterward.

- In an emergency when a Catholic priest is unavailable, baptism may be administered by anyone, regardless of their religious beliefs (see "Healing Rituals").

- Many Catholics attach importance to holy cards, statues, the crucifix, the rosary, or other items. Allowing the patient to keep these near their person can provide comfort.

- During some Catholic rituals, it is customary to sprinkle blessed water in the room or on the sick person. If this is contraindicated, the patient and family should be informed of this.

FOR MORE INFORMATION

Catholic Book Publishing Corporation. (1983). *Rites for ministry to the sick: Pastoral care of the sick, rites of anointing and viaticum.* Totowa, NJ: Author.

United States Catholic Conference. (2003). *The catechism of the Catholic Church* (CCC) 2nd ed. New York, NY: Doubleday.

CCC and other compendiums of Catholic Church doctrine are available online at http://www.vatican.va.

27 Seventh-Day Adventists

CONTRIBUTOR: *Mark Carr, PhD*

NURSE REVIEWER: *Rilla Taylor, EdD, RN*

Theology and Social History

The Seventh-Day Adventist (SDA) movement traces its history to the early 1840s. During these years, many persons of different Christian denominations, primarily in the United States, became convinced that Christ's second coming was imminent. This wondrously good news infused believers with hope and excitement, and many put their earthly affairs in order. From study of the biblical books of Daniel and Revelation, William Miller and his followers accepted that around October 22, 1844, Jesus would return. When Christ did not come on that date, many of the disappointed believers became disillusioned. One group of "Millerites," however, remained convicted of Christ's soon coming and deepened their study to determine where the calculations and assumptions could have been inaccurate. They subsequently learned of the seventh-day Sabbath from Seventh-Day Baptists. Following a short time of thinking that God was done trying to reach others with the Gospel message, they changed course and began aggressive outreach urging others to believe in the seventh-day Sabbath and second coming of Jesus.

A handful of key leaders shaped these early days. Joseph Bates, a Christian seaman and community leader joined together with Ellen and James White to lead the beleaguered group of Millerites. James was a pastor of the Christian Connection church with some measure of experience, but Ellen G. White brought the charisma of a young person moved by God's spirit. Viewed by many in Seventh-Day Adventism as a prophet of God, Ellen, along with her husband James and Joseph Bates, facilitated the transition from Millerism to a fully developed church. To incorporate their printed evangelistic efforts and bring structure to their growing numbers, they formally became the "Seventh-Day Adventist" church in 1864.

Since then, the church has grown to approximately 18 million members with the vast majority (around 93%) living outside the United States. The driving force of this church remains primarily focused on an evangelistic effort to share God's end time message of Sabbath keeping in anticipation of Jesus' second coming.

Deity/God or Ultimate Other

SDAs are monotheists, believing that there is one, triune God. Adventists recognize the same Yahweh God of the Hebrew bible and believe that the Jesus of the "New Testament" is the Christ or the promised Messiah spoken of in the Hebrew bible (Old Testament). It is integral to SDA faith that Jesus Christ (God incarnate) was then, and remains today, interested in the personal lives of every person. God is intimately personal, involved, and compassionate. God cares. The concept of God as being always present and aware is comforting, reassuring, and supportive. Although God is not bound by anthropomorphic tendencies, Adventists typically refer to God using masculine pronouns.

Views on Health and Well-Being

SDAs have always focused a great deal of attention on being healthy. In fact, early in SDA history, the church was shaped by what is known as "The Health Message." Theologically, the idea is that if we are healthy in heart and mind, we will have the opportunity to have as close a relationship with God as is possible. Furthermore, we will be more independent, productive, and able to serve others. Exercise, wearing healthful clothing, diet that excludes stimulants and the "unclean" meats listed in the Old Testament, sunshine, clean air, and sufficient rest are all seen as contributors to good health. Positive family relationships, all of whom are ideally in a relationship with God, also promote health and well-being.

Explanations for Disease and Illness

There is a fair measure of diversity in how SDAs may explain disease. Some will attribute disease and illness to God, believing that God either causes or allows persons to go through such difficulties as a means of drawing them closer to God-self, or to help them grow character. Most, however, attribute such things as disease and illness to the evil realities of this sin-affected world. If the bad things persons experience are to be blamed on the devil and evil, any and all good things that might evolve from such difficulties are attributed to God and His loving grace.

The Nature of Suffering and How to Address It

Suffering does not occur because God would want us to suffer (e.g., to punish, to purify, or test persons). Rather, suffering comes from the work of evil (impersonally put), or the evil one (Devil). Suffering is temporary given that God is involved and interested in relieving our plight with His love and care through Jesus and His community (body of Christ or the church). Meaning is found when remembering God's promise to connect with us and deliver us from the machinations of the evil one—"in the world to come if not this one." Hence, SDAs may find some comfort in reminders that suffering will end at the second advent. They often are heard to say, "This too shall pass."

Death, Dying, and Afterlife

Death is like sleep. Interpreting the creation story in the biblical book of Genesis, we believe that God "breathed into" humankind the "breath of life." At death, this breath goes back to God. Persons who have given themselves to God will not regain consciousness until the Second Coming of Jesus. Immortal life is a gift of God which we look forward to and believe we have. Yet, persons do not presently possess an eternal soul. One's eternal life is completely dependent upon God's gracious choice, which God gifts to persons after earthly life. The most comforting thing we might teach is that God is gracious toward us!

Quick and Condensed Definitions of Terms

Sabbath—Seventh day of the week (Saturday), observed as a holy day from sundown Friday evening to sundown Saturday.

Prayer

SDAs communicate with God/Jesus primarily through formal and informal prayer. SDAs often think of prayer as conversation with a Friend and use a colloquial style. Many SDAs also fast and meditate in an effort to draw closer to God. Corporate prayer life is primarily in the form of a pastoral prayer during worship services. SDAs actively pray for others, including local church members, societal leaders, and the "lost" (those who have not given their hearts to God) all over the world. Although some SDAs prefer praying on their knees, there is no official prescriptive about prayer posture.

Religious Calendar

Other than the weekly Sabbath, SDAs do not have holy days. Although most SDAs do enjoy the festivities of societal holidays such as Easter and Christmas, these holidays are not considered "holy days."

Health-Promoting Practices

SDAs are encouraged to avoid eating meat and opt for a vegetarian diet. Many, perhaps most, SDAs are lacto-ovo-vegetarians. SDAs who do eat meat likely will avoid "unclean" meats listed in Leviticus. Any food with porcine products is avoided. For the same reason, only seafood with fins and scales are acceptable. There is a fairly strong taboo against consumption of any alcoholic drink, caffeine, smoking, and use of drugs for nonmedical benefit. Health-promotion education offered in an SDA context will typically extol exercise, sunshine, trust in Divine Power, hydration, rest, vegetarian diet, and abstinence from abusive drugs. Rest is indeed an important aspect of Sabbath keeping. During the 24 hours of Sabbath, SDAs refrain from unnecessary work and study. Instead, they typically choose some form of corporate worship, fellowship with family or church members, spiritually nurturing activity, re-creation in nature, or service for others.

Healing Rituals

SDA ministers are occasionally asked by sick persons to provide an "anointing." The minister brings a small amount of olive oil and places a few drops of it on the patient's head. Then the minister, and perhaps a lay leader ("elder") from the congregation, will lay hands on the patient (i.e., touch the shoulder or head) praying that God will heal the patient— spiritually, if not physically or emotionally.

Other Unique Religious Beliefs, Rites, and Practices Related to Health or Illness

None.

Unique Religious Beliefs, Rites, and Practices Related to Birthing

Although not codified, SDAs generally circumcise male babies, often on the eighth day after birth in keeping with Mosaic law (i.e., the law given by God to Moses and presently observed by orthodox Jews).

Unique Religious Beliefs, Rites, or Practices Related to Childrearing

Traditional SDAs try to have morning and evening worship together as a family. This typically involves reading a devotional story or bible reading. Prayer is also an essential part of this worship time. It is thought that such time together when the children are young will instill positive habits in the children that will serve them well into adulthood. Children often attend Sabbath School prior to Sabbath morning church services. SDA children may attend a denominationally operated church school, academy, or university.

Unique Beliefs, Practices, and Rituals Surrounding Dying, Death, and Bereavement

North American SDAs observe death practices like those typically found in other Christian denominations in their locality. SDAs who have immigrated from other countries may have practices that mirror their culture of origin more.

Role of Religious Community (Persons or Organizations) During Health Challenges

Adventists have regular weekly worship services on Saturday (Sabbath) mornings. Sabbath School, a time of Bible study (typically from a lesson guide published by the church), is followed by the worship service, which is characteristically traditional Protestant nonliturgical style. No lectionary is followed, so worship themes and styles vary widely. Roughly half of SDA congregations will also have a midweek "prayer meeting."

Health promotion activities have traditionally been the purview of a church appointed "Health and Temperance Committee." Internationally, the church owns and operates about 170 hospitals, 440 clinics, 40 nursing homes, and numerous educational institutions for training nurses and other health care professionals. The church also runs the Adventist Development and Relief Agency that responds to disasters and introduces initiatives to improve hygiene, health, education, and so forth. Although a few congregations may have a parish nurse, it is more likely that the needs of the ill and indigent are addressed by deaconesses (elected, untrained women in the church), or in larger congregations, a "Dorcas Society" (also known as an Adventist Community Services Center, which offers its services to nonmembers as well). If a church member requests help or there is a death in a family, these deaconesses typically will support by bringing food and showing interest.

Role of Clergy During Health Challenges

The local pastor is expected to visit the sick. Many large congregations with multipastor staffs have a pastor solely devoted to visitation of members, including those who are ill. A pastoral visit typically will end with a prayer. When a patient requests anointing, the pastor, lay leader/s, and possibly close friends will plan a time for this special service (see "Healing Rituals").

Unique Religious Aspects of Family Involvement

SDAs are encouraged to not be "unequally yoked." That is, more traditional members still encourage their children to marry someone who shares SDA beliefs. Many SDAs, however, are not married to a SDA. Regardless, marriage is a sacred covenant. Sexual relations are to be reserved as an expression of love only in marriage.

Nursing Implications Unique to This Religious Tradition

- Given SDA beliefs regarding the "state of the dead" (i.e., death is sleep), statements that many Christians find comforting will be inappropriate (e.g., "Your loved one is looking down on you" or "Your loved is in

Heaven now"). Rather, an SDA is comforted by reminders that their loved one will awake one day when the Lord returns, that the hope of Heaven is sure.

- Consider the type of diet an SDA eats when planning care. While some may be vegans or lacto-ovo-vegetarian, others (especially immigrants and more liberal members) may eat meat. Unclean foods (e.g., pork) are not eaten. Porcine and shellfish products for medicinal or therapeutic purposes are typically treated as exceptions.

- Discuss with a SDA who is receiving health care on a Sabbath how that Sabbath can remain a time of rest and worship. They will likely accept necessary treatments and procedures but appreciate a more peaceful environment if it is possible.

- A very conservative SDA may have some hesitancy about accepting intimate health care from a clinician of the opposite gender.

FOR MORE INFORMATION

Visit http://www.adventist.org/

Schwarz, R. W. (1979). *Light bearers to the remnant*. Mountain View, CA: Pacific Press Publishing Association.

Taylor, E. J. & Carr, M. F. (2009). Nursing ethics in the Seventh-day Adventist religious tradition. *Nursing Ethics, 16,* 707–718.

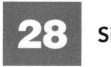 **Sikhs**

CONTRIBUTOR: *Pashaura Singh, PhD*

REVIEWERS: *Savitri W. Singh-Carlson, PhD, RN, and Harjit Kaur, MSocSc*

Theology and Social History

Sikhism is an independent religion, based upon the teachings of its founder Guru Nanak (1469–1539) and his nine successors. The Punjabi word *Sikh* means "disciple." People who identify themselves as Sikhs are disciples of *Akal Purakh* ("Timeless Being," God), the ten Sikh Gurus, and the sacred scripture called the *Adi Granth* (AG; "Original Book") or the *Guru Granth Sahib.*

The youngest of India's indigenous religions, Sikhism emerged in the Punjab province of north India five centuries ago. It quickly distinguished itself from the region's other religious traditions in its doctrines, practices, and orientations—away from ascetic renunciation and toward active engagement with the world. Although the Sikh scripture (*Guru Granth Sahib*) is universalistic in its teachings, Sikhism has, for the most part, been followed by the regional linguistic–cultural group known as the Punjabis. Religion remains highly important in the formation of group identity among the diasporic Sikh communities.

Sharing a history of British colonialism with other Indian religions, Sikhs have tended to migrate to the United Kingdom and former British colonies in East Africa, North America, and Australia. The Sikh diaspora was motivated initially by the annexation of Sikh territory into the British Raj, as well as economic reasons. As a largely traditional, sometimes semiliterate, rural group, diasporic Sikhs face a remarkable transition as they relocate to urban modern societies. Family relations and community honor tend to be sustained through the *gurdwara* (sites of communal worship and gathering). External symbols of the religion (e.g., turbans, beards) are often held to as visible markers of Sikh identity for young and old alike, although successive generations are redefining religious affiliation and cultural identity. Many Sikhs in the diaspora are less observant of external symbols, although they maintain their faith in the teachings of the Gurus. There is a clear distinction between the Khalsa (baptized Sikhs) and nonbaptized ones. For Khalsa Sikhs, the five Ks are core to their religious practice constituting the Rahit Maryada. Some nonbaptized Sikhs may have some or all of the five Ks as they align their practice with the religion.

Deity/God or Ultimate Other

Sikh religion is theistic. It believes in One God (*Akal Purukh*, "Timeless Being") who, as the creator and sustainer of the universe, watches over it lovingly as a parent. Like a father, he runs the world with justice, destroys evil, and supports good; like a mother, she is the source of love and grace and responds to the devotion of her humblest followers. Simultaneously "Father, Mother, Friend and Brother" (AG 168), God is without gender. *Akal Purakh* is constantly concerned with the personal life of the individual. Humans communicate with the divine Person through prayer and meditation on the divine Name (*nam simran*).

Views on Health and Well-Being

Sikhs view health and well-being as an asset of life. Human life is the most delightful experience with the gift of a healthy body. Indeed, a human being is called the epitome of creation in Sikhism: "All other creation is subject to you, O man/woman; you reign supreme on this earth." Although the existence of physical deformity and ugliness in the world is sometimes explained as the result of previous *karma*, it is intended for a higher divine purpose, which is beyond human comprehension.

Explanations for Disease and Illness

The notion of karma and rebirth is important for Sikh patients because they may believe that their illness results from the sins of previous lives. Each person is repeatedly reborn so that his or her soul may be ultimately purified and eventually join the divine cosmic consciousness.

Guru Nanak proclaimed: "When one indulges in carnal pleasures by forgetting God, then one's body contracts many ailments, punishing the wicked mind" (AG 1256). Human agents are responsible for their miserable condition. Sikhs are guided to maintain a balance by attending to the care of the physical and spiritual body. The balance of the mind, body, and spirit to attain health is achieved by adhering to the principles of *nam simran* and the recitation of the *banis* (daily prayers) for daily cleansing of the mind, daily showers in the ambrosial hour for cleansing the physical body, and participation in *seva* (voluntary service).

The Nature of Suffering and How to Address It

Guru Nanak diagnosed different types of suffering (*dukkh*) such as pang of separation from the divine beloved, pain of starvation, anguish of tyranny and death, affliction of bodily ailments, and torment of mental and spiritual diseases. All these pains, in fact, make suffering universal. They highlight different aspects of spiritual, mental, and physical suffering. Indeed, Guru Nanak acknowledges two levels of suffering, one which is innate to all human beings by virtue of their entanglement in the cycle of existence (*sansar*) and the other which is encountered in everyday life as a result of hunger, distress, tyranny, and so on. He proclaimed that the "whole world is groaning in suffering." In fact, suffering is an inevitable part of the human situation. To wish it were not there is to be oblivious of the divine Order (*hukam*): "Nanak, idle it is for one to ask for pleasure when pain comes. Pleasure and pain are like robes which one must wear as they come." Thus, suffering is not some kind of "illusion," but a stark reality of life. However, this does not mean that Sikh patients do not take pain medicine to ameliorate their suffering. While taking medicine, they do allow the experience of suffering to test or strengthen their will to live in high spirits (*chardi kala*).

Death, Dying, and Afterlife

Persons' actions in life determine their fate. For a dedicated Sikh, death is a joy to be welcomed when it comes, for it means the perfecting of his or her union with *Akal Purukh* ("Timeless Being") and a final release from the cycle of rebirth. For a self-willed person, by contrast, death means the culmination of his or her separation from the Divine and perpetuation of the process of reincarnation. The recitation of the scriptural hymns from the *Guru Granth Sahib* typically comforts a dying person. At the final moment, all are treated with respect, as no one is capable of making any judgment about whether one was a dedicated Sikh or not.

Quick and Condensed Definitions of Terms

Akal Purukh—"Timeless Being," God.

Granthi—Local spiritual leader, trained in the reading of Sikh scripture and other rituals; although custodians of gurdwaras, they are not ordained like clergy.

Gurdwara—Site of communal worship and gathering.

Guru Granth Sahib—or *Adi Granth* ("Original Book"), sacred scripture.

Khalsa Sikh—Sikhs who are baptized; they abide by the *Rahit* (code of conduct), which enjoinders them, among other things, to wear five items of external identity known from their Punjabi names as the five Ks. To become a Khalsa Sikh is a personal choice when one is ready for the Khalsa discipline, a decision often made late in life.

Sikh Rahit Maryada—Code of Conduct held as core to the faith for all Sikhs; however, the Khalsa Sikhs are stricter in their observance of the

Rahit. The *Rahit Maryada* is a commitment of a Khalsa Sikh and is taken as a vow when a Sikh partakes in the Amrit ceremony to be baptized.

Five Ks—These are unshorn hair (*kesh*), a wooden comb (*kanga*), a miniature sword (*kirpan*, literally this word is the combination of *"kirpa"* and *"an,"* meaning "grace" and "self-respect"), an iron "wrist-ring" (*kara*), and a pair of short breeches (*kachh*). A non-Khalsa Sikh may wear these as well.

Prayer

Prayer is an integral part of the Sikh tradition. It is both individual and corporate. For a Sikh, prayers are the recitation of *banis* (daily prayers) and *kirtan* (the singing of hymns from *Guru Granth Sahib*). Sikhs have a daily practice of rising in the ambrosial hour to shower and recite *nam simran* and the five *banis*, before having breakfast. In the evening at dusk, Sikhs recite *Rehraas Sahib*, and before retiring to bed, the Sikh recites *Kirtan Sohila*. Before reciting prayers, Sikhs wash their hands, do a mouthwash, remove any footwear, cover their head with a turban or scarf (for women) and sit to recite them. At the end of their prayers, Sikhs stand up to recite the *Ardas*.

Religious Calendar

The most important festival day in Sikh calendar is Baisakhi (Vaisakhi) Day, which usually falls on April 13. Celebrated throughout India as New Year's Day, it has been considered the birthday of the Sikh community ever since Guru Gobind Singh inaugurated the Khalsa on Baisakhi Day in 1699. Sikhs also celebrate the autumn festival of lights, Divali, as the day when Guru Hargobind was released from imprisonment under the Mughal emperor Jahangir. Harimandir Sahib (Golden Temple) in Amritsar is illuminated for the occasion. Guru Gobind Singh added a third festival of Hola Mahalla (March/April), which is celebrated with military exercises and various athletic and literary contests. The anniversaries of the births and deaths of the Gurus are marked by the "unbroken reading" (*akhand path*) of the entire Sikh scripture by a team of readers over a period of roughly 48 hr. Such occasions are called *Gurpurbs* ("holidays associated with the Gurus"). The birthdays of Guru Nanak (usually in November) and Guru Gobind Singh (December/January) and the martyrdom days of Guru Arjan (May/June) and Guru Tegh Bahadur (November/December), in particular, are celebrated around the world.

Health-Promoting Practices

The Adi Granth does not prescribe any dietary rules. Generally, it lays emphasis on "consuming only those foods which do not cause pain in the body or breed evil thoughts in the mind" (AG, 16). Most of the Punjabi Sikhs show a healthy and approved appetite for simple vegetables and milk products. Their favorite choice is the diet of "corn bread and mustard greens" (*makki di roti* and *sag*) with buttermilk (*lassi*). They also eat rice and flat wheat bread (*chapati*), supplemented by a lentil curry (*dal*) and other vegetables. Khalsa Sikhs are strict vegetarians, often consuming milk and cheese but not eggs. The diet for nonbaptized Sikhs can be either vegetarians or nonvegetarian.

The *Sikh Rahit Maryada* cautiously permits the eating of *jhataka* meat (killed with a single blow). Most importantly, food served in the "community kitchens" (*langars*) of gurdwaras is exclusively vegetarian. In order to keep the egalitarian emphasis of the Gurus, the serving of eggs and meat is not permitted in the community kitchen. The use of tobacco and other nonmedicinal drugs is strictly prohibited to the Khalsa Sikhs. Similarly, the consumption of alcohol is forbidden for all Sikhs.

Healing Rituals

None.

Other Unique Religious Beliefs, Rites, and Practices Related to Health or Illness

Khalsa Sikhs (both men and women) are prohibited from four gross sins: cutting the hair, using tobacco, committing adultery, and eating meat.

Unique Religious Beliefs, Rites, and Practices Related to Birthing

There are no beliefs with regard to special disposal of afterbirth. In the Sikh tradition, circumcision is strictly prohibited.

Unique Religious Beliefs, Rites, or Practices Related to Childrearing

When the mother and the child are released from the hospital, they are taken to the local *gurdwara* for thanksgiving and prayers. The child is given a new name through a religious ceremony by the *Granthi* who seeks the first letter of the name by opening the Sikh scripture at random.

Unique Beliefs, Practices, and Rituals Surrounding Dying, Death, and Bereavement

No rituals (derived from other religious traditions or of any other origins) should be performed when a Sikh dies in the hospital. The *Sikh Rahit Maryada* explicitly states that "a dying person should not be taken from his bed and placed on the ground." It is common practice for family members to recite Guru Arjan's *Sukhmani* or other hymns from the Adi Granth in the presence of a dying person. These devotional hymns are accessible on compact disk and can be played in the absence of a family member. When a Sikh dies, the *Kirtan Sohila* is recited.

In the case of the death of a Khalsa Sikh, the five Ks should be left on the dead body. Even if any of these five items (such as *kirpan*) were removed at the time of surgery, they should be restored on the body of the deceased. The hair should be neatly tied in a knot over the head (in the case of male Sikhs) and covered with a small turban. The health care workers will earn the gratitude of family members if they are sensitive to these traditions. Moreover, it is always helpful to talk to the patients beforehand about specific instructions that they would like carried out in the event of their death.

Role of Religious Community (Persons or Organizations) During Health Challenges

The congregational worship takes place in the local *gurdwara* where the main focus is upon the *Guru Granth Sahib,* installed ceremoniously every morning. It consists mainly of the singing of scriptural passages set to music with the accompaniment of instruments. This singing of hymns (*kirtan*) in a congregational setting is the heart of the Sikh devotional experience. Through such *kirtan,* the devotees attune themselves to vibrate in harmony with the divine Word, which has the power to transform and unify their consciousness. The exposition of the scriptures, known as *katha* ("homily"), may be delivered at an appropriate time during the service by the *granthi* of the gurdwara or by the traditional Sikh scholar (*giani*). At the conclusion of the service, all who are present will join in reciting the *Ardas* ("Petition," the Sikh Prayer) that invokes the divine grace and recalls the common rich heritage of the community. Then follows the reading of the *vak* ("divine command") and the distribution of *karah prashad* ("sanctified food") to everyone. In the diaspora, regular religious gathering takes place in gurdwaras every Sunday. Members of Sikh faith frequently offer prayers for others who are ill.

Local community social service is made possible through the *gurdwaras.* A Sikh community may band together to support a community health organization (e.g., raise funds for a hospital) or to offer support to a member family with a seriously ill member.

Role of Clergy During Health Challenges

Religious leaders such as *Granthis* (Readers) at the *Gurdwara* offer *Ardas* ("Petition," Sikh Prayer) for members of the tradition who are ill. They also visit the Sikh patients with the family members to offer prayers with them in their presence.

Unique Religious Aspects of Family Involvement

The parents, siblings, children, and other distant relatives are generally quite involved when a family member becomes ill. Often they participate collaboratively in health care decision making for their loved one. They also provide support by offering prayers.

Nursing Implications Unique to This Religious Tradition

- With Sikh patients, inquire if they are baptized Sikh (Khalsa). Baptized Sikhs will uphold the *Rahit Maryada* code of conduct, which prescribes several behaviors about which nurses should know. In addition to the five Ks, the baptized and observant Sikh will refrain from meat, alcohol, and other stimulants; remain celibate until marriage and then be monogamous; volunteer to serve humanity; hold women with respect (e.g., not have a man conduct an intimate physical assessment on a woman); and meditate and pray daily.

- The daily prayers can be read from the *Gutka*, a small book of prayers that Khalsa Sikhs will typically always carry on their person. This book should be handled with utmost cleanliness. Prior to reading the prayer book, a Sikh will want to cleanse himself/herself—by washing hands, rinsing mouth, removing footwear (if possible). They will want to sit up to recite the prayers if possible. Sikh patients can meditate on the divine Name by themselves if they are conscious enough. The "remembrance of the divine Name" is the means of liberation from all types of suffering in the world.

- Whether baptized or not as Sikh, many observe the five Ks, which are vital symbols of Sikh identity (i.e., wearing unshorn hair, sword, shorts, comb, wrist ring). These five Ks should be respected by not being removed from the patient unless absolutely necessary. Discuss with the patient and family how best to respect these symbols while delivering health care. For example, the *kirpan* (sword) may be kept ordinarily but may be removed at the time of surgery. The shaving of hair for the purpose of surgery is permitted, but must be discussed with the patient and family. There have been incidents where RNs have cut the beard of a Sikh without permission, motivating the patient to martyr himself within 24 hours because of this breech of spiritual or moral conduct.

- A patient from the Sikh tradition might desire to listen to a CD of devotional singing (*kirtan*) of hymns from the *Guru Granth Sahib* to uplift his heart, mind, and soul. A nurse can arrange with the help of the family to play such a CD for the patient.

- A nurse might support the patient if he or she wants to attend the congregational worship at the local *gurdwara*.

FOR MORE INFORMATION

Visit http://www.sikhnet.com, http://www.sikhchic.com, or http://www.sikhs.org

Singh, N. K. (2011). *Sikhism: An introduction*. London, UK: Tauris.

Singh, P. (2010). Sikh traditions. In W. G. Oxtoby & R. C. Amore (Eds.), *World religions: Eastern tradition* (3rd ed., pp. 106–143). Don Mills, Ontario: Oxford University Press.

Unitarian Universalists

CONTRIBUTOR: *The Reverend Susan Ritchie, PhD*

NURSE REVIEWER: *Kathe Kelly, BSN, RN, OCN*

Theology and Social History

Unitarian Universalism is the result of the 1961 consolidation of two liberal Protestant traditions. Although Unitarianism had its origins in 16th century Eastern Europe, the numbers of Unitarians outside of the United States are now quite small. Unitarianism in North America emerged as an early 19th century split within the Congregational Church. Interested in human capacity for growth and development, and confident in the powers of human reason, Unitarians placed high value on education and social progress.

Universalism arose as a progressive, grassroots movement in 18th century New England. Unitarians stressed the positive aspects of humanity, which they contrasted to what they thought was an excessive focus on original sin and human depravity in other Protestant traditions. Universalists historically stressed the benevolence of God and derived their name from the doctrine of universal salvation, which held that a loving God would not condemn anyone to eternal punishment in hell. Both traditions placed high values on democratic process and personal freedom and stressed the inherent worth and dignity of all people.

Today, Unitarian Universalism is a noncreedal faith that has extended beyond its Christian roots to explore the ethical and spiritual value of teachings from other religions and also secular sources. Congregations are organized along democratic and nonhierarchical principles. The first denomination to ordain women as well as openly gay and lesbian persons to the ministry, most Unitarian Universalists (UUs) identify with liberal and progressive social values. In keeping with its historic roots, the tradition tends to attract well-educated persons from the middle and upper middle classes (even as diversity in membership is valued).

Deity/God or Ultimate Other

Both Unitarianism and Universalism were historically Christian, with a corresponding understanding of God. The teachings of Jesus were considered an important guide to ethical and moral life, but both traditions questioned the divinity of Jesus early on. Because Unitarian Universalism is a noncreedal faith, current members hold diverse theological understandings on the question of God. Some hold to a traditional Christian theism, some identify as humanists, and some draw their understanding of the holy from other traditions (e.g., Buddhism, earth-based religions).

Views on Health and Well-Being

UUs embrace a holistic and scientifically based understanding of mental, spiritual, and physical health.

Explanations for Disease and Illness

Unitarian Universalism sees no conflict between science and religion and would not make an explanation for disease outside of a scientific one. UU patients tend to take comfort in being educated as fully as possible about the medical understanding of their diseases.

The Nature of Suffering and How to Address It

UUs see suffering as a natural component of all human life and not as the result of divine displeasure or human sin. UUs feel that the social and physical causes of suffering are best remedied through the progressive actions of compassionate people. Unlikely to see suffering as having an inherent meaning, UUs nonetheless are likely to look for how their personal tragedy might result in good for others. UUs are often interested in organ donation, for example, and in clinical trials that might advance scientific understanding.

Death, Dying, and Afterlife

Being theologically diverse, individual UUs hold a wide array of beliefs about death. They may believe in a traditional Christian heaven, in no afterlife at all, or in a conception of life after death drawn from eclectic or nonwestern sources. UUs take comfort in the idea that one's good deeds and more positive influences live on in the lives of the people they have touched. UUs believe that death is best understood in its natural context as the inevitable conclusion of all life, and as such, is not to be feared.

Quick and Condensed Definitions of Terms

UUs prefer gender inclusive and secular language. A nonverbalized "term" is a flame within a chalice that is often the symbol of the UU faith; this may be worn as jewelry.

Prayer

There is no proscription about how, when, or what to pray. UU congregations and individuals may engage in prayer, meditation, silent contemplation, worship, and other types of spiritual practice. It is customary in most congregations to acknowledge the struggles of individuals during the course of worship. This can occur in a variety of ways (e.g., through a prayer, spoken or silent sharing, lighting candles, or other practices reflecting a congregation's traditions). Clergy may or may not offer to pray with ill persons depending on that individual's preferences.

Religious Calendar

UUs typically observe Christmas, Easter, and sometimes Jewish holidays, both within their families and in worship. Observance, however, is flexible and not strictly proscribed. It is also freely mixed with more secular understandings of the holidays.

Health-Promoting Practices

There are no proscriptions. However, as UUs stress personal responsibility, educate themselves about health, and trust educated professionals, they tend to be highly compliant and motivated when recommended health-promoting therapies, disciplines, or lifestyle changes.

Healing Rituals

There are no specific healing rituals.

Other Unique Religious Beliefs, Rites, and Practices Related to Health or Illness

None.

Unique Religious Beliefs, Rites, and Practices Related to Birthing

None. Many, but not all, UUs are interested in natural childbirth.

Unique Religious Beliefs, Rites, or Practices Related to Childrearing

None, although UUs tend to be interested in progressive and positive childrearing philosophies.

Unique Beliefs, Practices, and Rituals Surrounding Dying, Death, and Bereavement

No specific rituals. UUs typically, but not always, prefer a memorial service that is a celebration of the uniqueness of the deceased person to a funeral with a body present. Many UUs are interested in cremation, or other innovative practices, such as environmentally friendly burials.

Role of Religious Community (Persons or Organizations) During Health Challenges

There is Sunday morning worship of about an hour in length, with readings, music, news of the community, and a sermon or message. Other than the act of gathering itself, the sermon is often central.

All support systems are based in local congregations and vary across congregations. In congregations with professional clergy, the clergy are expected to coordinate support efforts. Many congregations have pastoral care associates or a "Caring Committee" to support members in situations requiring extra support and care. These members may make pastoral calls. It is always appropriate to ask the local congregation's minister about such resources directly.

Role of Clergy During Health Challenges

It is the role of the clergy (ministers) to visit the sick in the congregation. Patients may or may not, however, desire to speak with a UU minister. (Likewise, some may and some may not choose to speak with a hospital chaplain.)

Unique Religious Aspects of Family Involvement

Many people become UUs as adults and may not share their religions identification with their family of origin. There can be tensions resulting from religious difference because of this. UU patients may need and appreciate reassurance that their religious wishes, and not those of more conservative family members, will be respected.

Nursing Implications Unique to This Religious Tradition

- Many congregations make the Sunday morning sermon or message available in print or online; patients may appreciate having access to these.

- Perhaps because it is a small and noncreedal tradition, UUism is often misunderstood and even maligned. Such insensitivity and disrespect make it especially important to recognize that UUs like to know that their religious practices and values will be respected.

- Given some UUs would prefer no clergy or chaplain visit, it is important to ask what services or clergy the UU patient would welcome.

FOR MORE INFORMATION

Visit the Unitarian Universalist Association website: www.uua.org.

Buehrens, J., & Church, F. (1998). *Chosen faith: An introduction to Unitarian universalism.* Boston, MA: Beacon Press.

Index